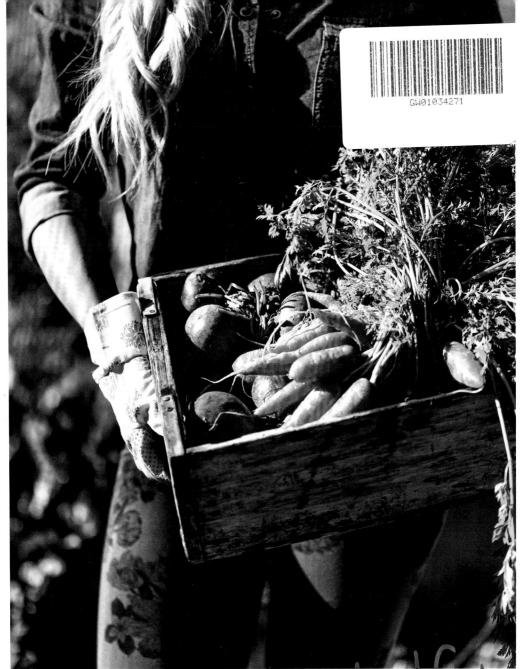

Mindful
EATING

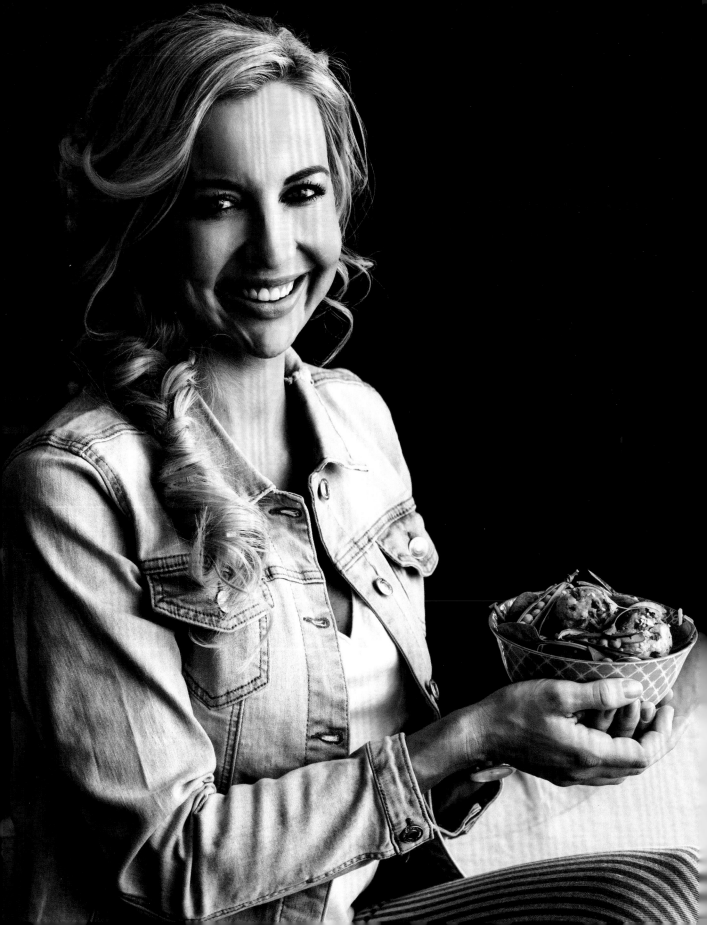

Dear Jeanette

For the ♡ of Healthy living!

Invest time in your health, it's the
Best investment you will ever make

♡e
Izelle
xxx.

Mindful
EATING

IZELLE HOFFMAN

PHOTOGRAPHY BY TOBY MURPHY

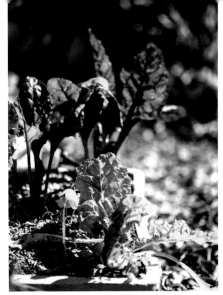
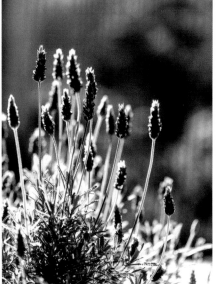
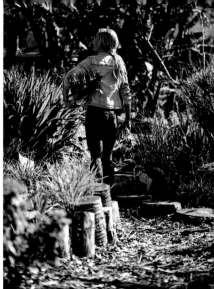

Published in 2020 by Struik Lifestyle, an imprint of
Penguin Random House South Africa (Pty) Ltd
Company Reg. No. 1953/000441/07
The Estuaries, 4 Oxbow Crescent, Century Avenue,
Century City 7441, Cape Town, South Africa
PO Box 1144, Cape Town, 8000, South Africa

www.penguinrandomhouse.co.za

PUBLISHER: Beverley Dodd
MANAGING EDITOR: Cecilia Barfield
EDITOR: Bronwen Maynier
DESIGNER: Helen Henn
PROOFREADER and INDEXER: Joy Nel
PHOTOGRAPHER: Toby Murphy
STYLIST: Brita du Plessis
ASSISTANTS: Anna-Mart Willemse from
    The Hurst Campus Culinary Academy,
    www.thehurstcampus.co.za and Phillipa Hill
MAKE-UP: Benecos SA
HAIR: Tamryn Botha Palladium Hair Co
CLOTHING: Freddy SA
STYLING: Natasha Human
JEWELLERY: Jenna Clifford

Reproduction: Hirt & Carter Cape (Pty) Ltd
Printing and binding: C&C Offset Printing Co., Ltd, China

ISBN 978-1-43231-052-3

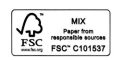

MIX
Paper from responsible sources
FSC™ C101537
FSC www.fsc.org

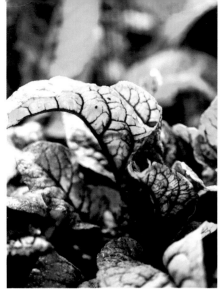
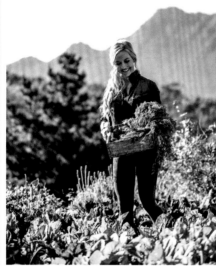
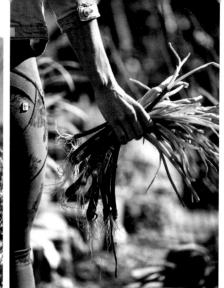

CONTENTS

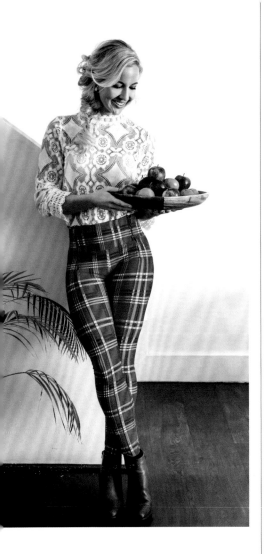

INTRODUCTION

This is not a cookbook; this is a 'change your perception of food' book!

Let's start with some food for thought ... for the LOVE of healthy living! My name is Izelle Hoffman and I am a lifestyle chef. What is a lifestyle chef, you ask? Someone who cooks according to their lifestyle, of course! I was born with congenital hip dysplasia. Fourteen operations later, I aim to make people aware of the health benefits of eating the right foods and choosing a life of health and wellness. I am differently abled, NOT disabled ... so what's your excuse?

I grew up on a farm just outside Bela-Bela, in Limpopo province. With a farmer for a dad and an amazing landscaper for a mom, my environment encouraged an interest in and understanding of food sources. Once you are aware of all the time and nurturing that goes into getting the perfect vegetable onto your plate, you appreciate and enjoy it so much more; you can almost taste the love and care. Growing vegetables and experimenting with different flavours was a part of my upbringing. With both grandmothers and my mother boasting world-class vegetable gardens, and an aunt who was the moderator of home economics for the North West province, my development into a 'conscious foodie' was inevitable!

Today I encourage people from all walks of life to rethink what they put into their bodies. Quality over quantity, always. Focus on the quality of your ingredients rather than how many ingredients you use when preparing a meal. And always start with the right ingredients. If you do, whatever you make will be a healthy masterpiece.

While I never formally trained as a chef, I grew up in a household where the majority of family time was spent in the kitchen or outside around the braai, preparing and cooking amazing food ... comfort food like goulash and potjie, festive food like roast chicken and leg of lamb, snack platters that still remind me of rugby on Saturdays and Christmas Eve with close family, and scrumptious baked goods that recall my aunt's visits from faraway

Rustenburg or my grandmothers' baking days, when all the grandchildren were invited.

In 1992, author Gary Chapman conceptualised the Five Love Languages: words of affirmation, acts of service, receiving gifts, quality time and physical touch. I think I speak all five of them! You see, preparing and cooking a meal for a loved one is my love language, and it involves every single one of Gary's Five Love Languages. Let me explain.

WORDS OF AFFIRMATION We all like to hear the following: 'Can I make you something to eat?' or 'I made a fresh batch of your favourite biscuits this morning; can I make us a cup of coffee, then you can tell me about your day?'

ACTS OF SERVICE Actions speak louder than words. Cooking a meal takes thought, time and effort. It's something I love doing, so I approach it with a positive attitude and keep the happiness of the person for whom I am cooking front of mind.

RECEIVING GIFTS That OMG moment. That 'I cannot believe this is healthy' moment. I always cook with these moments in mind, and when I get that reaction, I know the recipe is a keeper.

QUALITY TIME I love spending time in the kitchen, and then sharing a meal and taking a moment to appreciate the smile on someone's face while they eat my food. It's just the best! I firmly believe that some of the most cherished moments in life happen around the dinner table or over a meal, and that the value of this should never be underestimated.

PHYSICAL TOUCH I always say that a scrumptious, healthy meal and a hug go hand in hand. They both give you that feel-good fuzzy feeling in your tummy, that feeling of belonging and of being loved. Whether cooking for a loved one or for someone less fortunate, I cook with love. There's nothing better than getting stuck in and preparing a meal for those dear to me and close to my heart.

Be the difference you want to see in the world, and share the love (in my case, food and cooking) – the world needs more of that!

And remember: time and health are two of the most precious commodities, neither of which can be bought. Invest time in your health – it is the best investment you will ever make. I urge you to always strive to be the best version of yourself, not only for yourself, but also for your loved ones. Respect yourself enough to want the best health, and make the most of life.

As author and motivational speaker Jim Rohn once said, 'Take care of your body. It's the only place you have to live.'

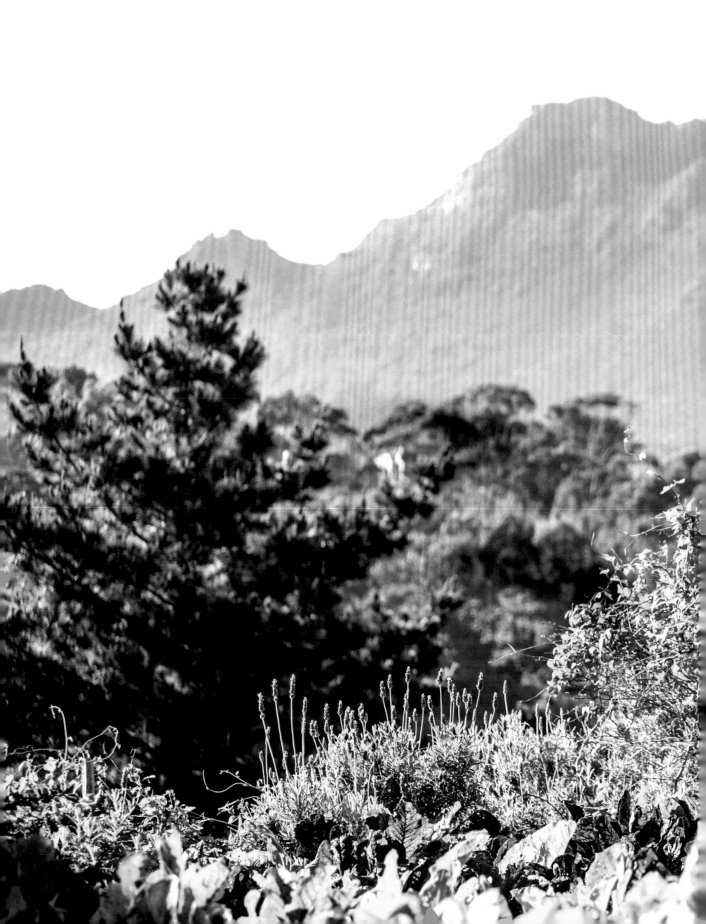

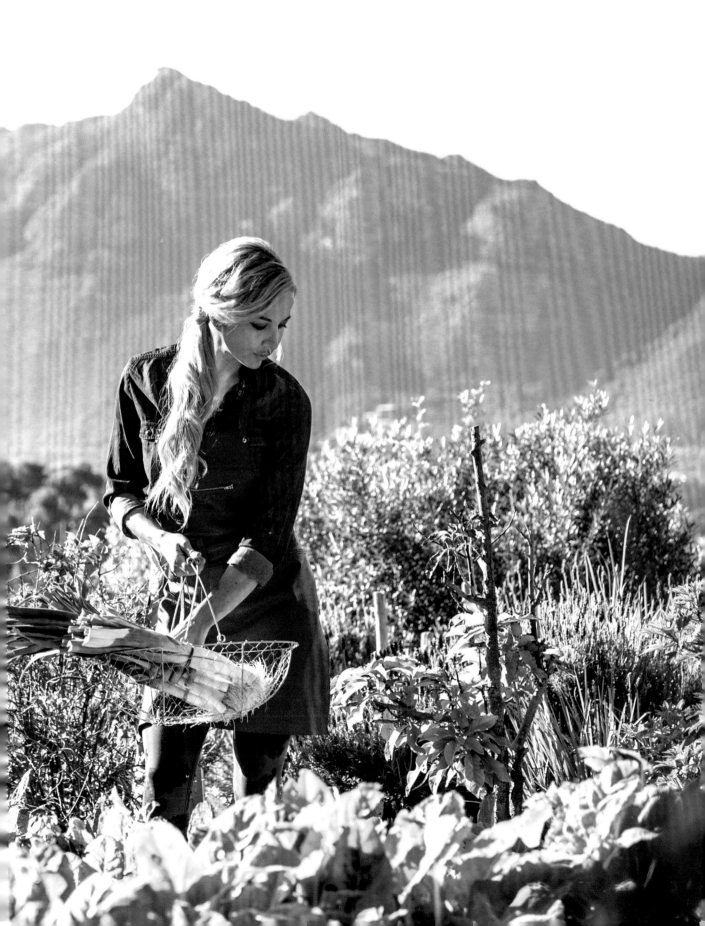

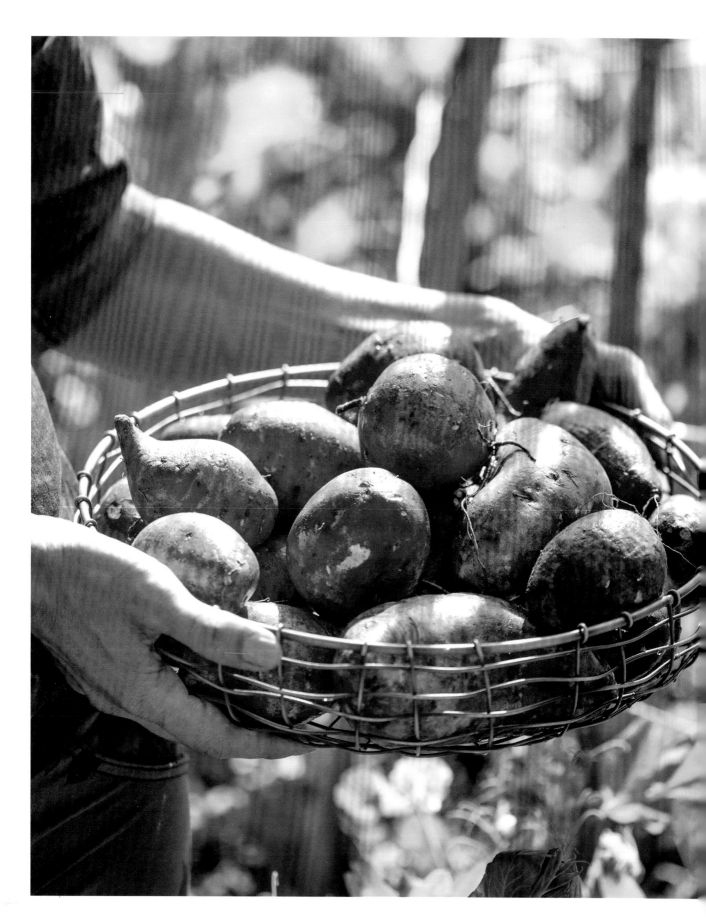

BEST FRIENDS FOR LIFE

... the good stuff

When it comes to my pantry, I have a few best friends I simply cannot live without. You know, those close friends who make all the difference in the world. Not only do they make you feel better, but also the impact they have on you (and your health) is seriously something to write a cookbook about!

Are you aware of what you eat? Do you ever turn a product over to read the list of ingredients before you consume it? Because if you don't know what you are eating, how can you control the effect it has on your health and wellness?

Here is a list of ingredients I always have at home, as well as a little information about each. I'm sharing it with love so that you can have the opportunity to become the best and healthiest version of yourself.

ALKALISING CITRUS Although themselves acidic, citrus fruits such as lemons and limes have an alkalising effect on the body. They are also loaded with vitamin C. Vitamin C content is always highest when the fruit is freshly cut. A squeeze of love in the shape of a lemon, who knew?

ALLSPICE This is derived from the dried, unripe berries of the *Pimenta dioica*, and delivers the flavours of many different spices, including cinnamon, cloves, nutmeg and pepper. Allspice is an anti-inflammatory, with antiseptic, antiviral and antifungal properties.

ALMONDS Whether in the form of milk, flour, butter or flakes, almonds are packed with nutritional benefits. They boost the immune system, help repair damaged skin, help prevent cancer, reduce the risk of osteoporosis and have alkalising properties. They are also a source of vitamin E, magnesium and high-quality protein.

APPLE CIDER VINEGAR This clever ingredient regulates the body's pH balance, detoxifies and reduces inflammation.

BALSAMIC VINEGAR Balsamic vinegar improves digestion, keeps the immune system strong and helps balance blood sugar levels.

BANANAS Not only are bananas anti-inflammatory, they are also one of those versatile fruits that can either be eaten as a snack on their own, frozen and added to smoothies or used in baking.

BICARBONATE OF SODA You will find this in my pantry as well as in the bathroom next to my toothbrush. Bicarbonate of soda alkalises the body, and so drinking half a teaspoon dissolved in water before I go to bed at night helps neutralise the acidity build-up of the day. It also provides relief from colds and flu, and supports healthy detoxification.

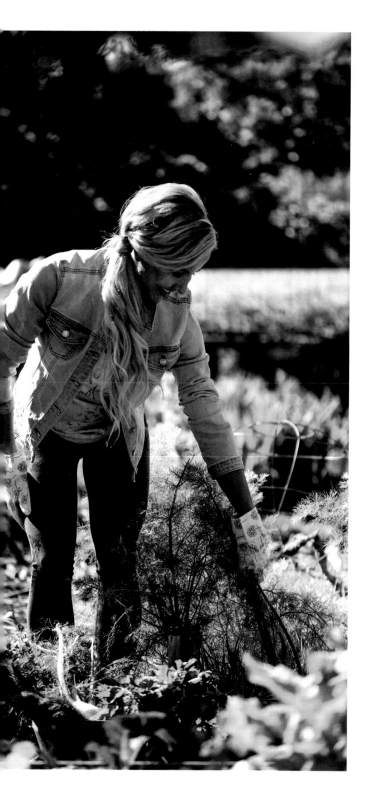

BLACK PEPPER Why do we add pepper to our food? When I ask this during cooking demonstrations, I always get the most interesting answers, but mostly people cannot tell me why they add pepper to their meals. My reason? It increases nutrient absorption and improves digestion, so you can get the most out of every meal, every time.

BLUEBERRIES AND BAOBAB POWDER Blueberries are one of the best antioxidant foods, second only to baobab powder. I always have frozen blueberries in the freezer and baobab powder in the pantry to bake blueberry crumble or make a nutritious breakfast smoothie.

BUCKWHEAT Anti-inflammatory, gluten free and easily digestible, buckwheat is beneficial in improving bone health and a rich source of fibre.

BUTTERBEANS Also known as lima beans, these gems are anti-inflammatory, assist in bone health, reduce arthritis, enhance sleep, detoxify the body and help with mineral absorption.

BUTTERNUT Butternut is an anti-inflammatory rich in slow-digesting carbohydrates and vitamin C, which makes it one of my favourite vegetables. It is also highly alkaline, lowers cholesterol and boosts immune function.

CANNELLINI BEANS Also known as white kidney beans, cannellinis are high in protein, rich in fibre and contain significant amounts of magnesium, which aids blood flow and is a natural way of maintaining artery health.

CAYENNE PEPPER Dr Schulze, one of the foremost authorities on natural healing and herbal medicine, says, 'If you master only one herb in your life, master cayenne pepper. It is more powerful than any other.' Cayenne pepper is an antiseptic, antifungal antihistamine that fights infections.

CHIA SEEDS A source of high-quality protein, chia seeds assist in digestive health because of their high fibre content, and maintain bone strength because of their high calcium content.

CHICKPEAS I love chickpeas, whether grilled and flavoured as a snack, served in a vegetarian curry or pulped and mixed with a few other ingredients to form the base of a cake. Chickpeas are a good source of fibre, rich in calcium, anti-inflammatory, and boost the immune system.

CHOCOLATE I keep a slab of locally made Gayleen's Decadence in my pantry, because it's preservative free, dairy free and sweetened with raw honey.

CINNAMON Cinnamon is loaded with antioxidants, lowers blood sugar levels and has a powerful anti-diabetic effect. It is anti-inflammatory, antiviral, antifungal and antibacterial.

CLOVES Cloves are anti-inflammatory, antibacterial and antimicrobial, and help treat digestive issues. They also preserve bone density and give relief from inflammation and pain.

CRANBERRIES Cranberries are rich in antioxidants, which flush toxins from the body, leading to improved digestion and metabolism. They are also anti-inflammatory and have a high fibre content. Be on the lookout for cranberries sweetened with pineapple juice instead of sugar.

DATES Dates are rich in selenium, manganese, copper and magnesium, all of which are required to keep bones healthy and prevent conditions such as osteoporosis.

ESSENCES Essences and essential oils can really add the wow factor to any meal, sometimes even in the most unexpected way. I mean, who knew the secret to the perfect balsamic cranberry glaze would be found in a teaspoon of caramel essence? (No kidding, see the recipe on page 142.) I always have caramel, vanilla and peppermint essences in my pantry.

FLAXSEEDS Flaxseeds are high in omega-3 and fibre. They are anti-inflammatory, antiviral, antifungal and antibacterial immune system boosters.

GARLIC Antiviral, antifungal and anti-inflammatory, garlic assists in detoxification and boosting the metabolism, and is a natural dewormer that kills parasites. I use both black and white fresh garlic, and keep dried garlic powder and flakes in my pantry.

GINGER My go-to reason for using ginger is that it relieves pain caused by arthritis, but it is also anti-inflammatory and antifungal, and boosts the immune system. I always have both fresh and dried ginger to hand. I also drink hot water with freshly grated ginger, lemon juice, raw honey and cayenne pepper to give my immune system that much-needed boost if I start feeling ill or a bit rundown.

GREEN BEANS 'Green fingers', as I call them, are full of dietary fibre and loaded with vitamin C. They improve bone health by preventing bone deterioration and osteoporosis, and boost the immune system.

HERBS I prefer fresh over dried, but I do love using a combination of both sometimes. I keep a store of the following fresh herbs in my garden or fridge and their dried versions in my pantry:
Basil is anti-inflammatory and antibacterial, strengthens the immune system and eliminates infections.
Coriander, also known as cilantro, is anti-inflammatory, antibacterial and antifungal.
Mint is one of my favourite herbs. Antibacterial, antifungal and anti-inflammatory, it improves digestion.
Parsley is so much more than just a garnish; it packs an unexpected nutritional punch. High in vitamins A and C and calcium, it is anti-inflammatory, improves bone health, is a blood purifier and boosts the immune system.
Rosemary is an anti-inflammatory, antibacterial immunity booster that helps liver detoxification and improves blood circulation.
Thyme boosts the immune system, is antiviral, antifungal and anti-inflammatory, and improves bone health.

LONG-STEM BROCCOLI Broccoli is a natural antibiotic, antiviral and alkaliser that is rich in calcium and fibre and improves immunity.

MUSTARD Mustard contains calcium, phosphorus, manganese and magnesium in sufficient amounts to make it highly beneficial for the development of strong bones. Because I am prone to osteoporosis, I try to include mustard in my diet on a weekly basis in the form of powder and seeds by making honey-mustard flavoured dishes or dressings. Mustard also assists in the reduction of intestinal inflammation and suppressing the appetite.

NON-STICK COOKING SPRAY I prefer an olive oil–based cooking spray (see 'olive oil' below).

NUTMEG Nutmeg is an anti-inflammatory antiseptic that helps treat joint pain and arthritis.

OLIVE OIL We all have our reasons why we prefer certain oils, but without a doubt my oil base of choice is olive oil, specifically for its amazing health benefits. Olive oil helps reduce inflammation and prevent osteoporosis, and is essential for bone health because it assists in the absorption of calcium and the mineralisation of bones, all of which are qualities I look for in a product, given my hip dysplasia and related joint pain.

ONIONS I prefer red onions for their slightly sweet taste and the burst of colour they add to dishes. Onions are a natural antibiotic and antiseptic, so are a big YES, especially in winter. They purify the blood, regulate blood sugar levels and improve digestion. They are also anti-inflammatory. In addition to fresh onions, in my pantry you will find dried onion powder and flakes.

ORYX DESERT SALT What is the purpose of adding salt during cooking? It's to enhance flavour, right? So why not start by using a good-quality salt to do the job? Sundried and unrefined with no additives will bring out the best in your food in the healthiest way possible.

PAPRIKA Smoked or sweet, paprika is antibacterial, anti-inflammatory and high in vitamin C. It helps ease arthritis and joint pain, and aids in iron and antioxidant absorption.

PECAN NUTS Pecan nuts contain various nutrients, minerals, antioxidants and vitamins, are anti-inflammatory, support the immune system and promote healthy digestion.

PINEAPPLE Pineapple must be my ultimate favourite fruit. Besides the fact that it is anti-inflammatory and reduces inflammation in joints and muscles, it also boosts immunity and improves blood circulation, which is another thing I am conscious about.

PUMPKIN SEEDS These are an alkalising anti-inflammatory with 32 g of plant-based protein per 100 g. They are rich in omega-3, zinc and sleep-promoting magnesium.

QUINOA Quinoa is called the complete plant-based protein because it contains all nine essential amino acids. Gluten free, with a low glycaemic index and very high in fibre, quinoa lowers cholesterol, helps prevent colon cancer and contributes to muscle formation.

RAW CACAO Raw cacao contains very high amounts of antioxidants, reduces appetite and helps with weight loss. It alleviates stress, helps manage depression and regulates blood pressure. It is a fantastic source of calcium too.

RAW HONEY Salt needs sweet and vice versa to enhance taste and flavour. So when you add sweetness, choose a sweetness that has a healing effect on your body and health. Raw honey is antiviral and antifungal, and contains powerful antioxidants. It helps ward off allergies, stabilise blood pressure and balance blood sugar levels. It also boosts the immune system and promotes digestive health.

ROSA TOMATOES Tomatoes help reduce inflammation, improve bone health and boost the immune system. I choose to cook with rosa tomatoes, because I find normal-sized tomatoes too watery and cherry tomatoes too sour. Rosa tomatoes are concentrated in taste, yet deliciously sweet, and are jam-packed with all the health benefits and goodness of regular tomatoes.

SESAME SEEDS Sesame seeds are anti-inflammatory and high in protein. They improve bone health, prevent osteoporosis and aid digestion.

SPINACH An anti-inflammatory high in fibre and antioxidants, spinach strengthens bones and helps the brain and nervous system function.

SWEET PEPPERS Sweet peppers are anti-inflammatory, loaded with antioxidants and a great source of immune system–boosting vitamin E. I always have pimiento and bell peppers in my fridge.

SWEET POTATO Sweet potato is an anti-inflammatory immune booster, full of nutrients and rich in beta-carotene (an important antioxidant and precursor to vitamin A). It also regulates blood sugar levels and is easily digestible because of its high fibre content.

TAMARI Tamari is a gluten-free soy sauce, which is slightly thicker and darker than regular soy sauce. In combination with raw honey it gives the wow factor to grilled salmon, but also creates a beautiful sticky marinade for beef strips and chicken fillets. Tamari contains niacin (vitamin B3), which helps with joint mobility and arthritis, aids in proper brain function and maintains skin health.

TURMERIC Curcumin is a natural anti-inflammatory compound found in turmeric that can be absorbed up to 2 000 per cent in combination with black pepper and/or an oil base such as olive oil. Turmeric also drastically increases the antioxidant capacity of the body and optimises function of the liver, the body's primary organ of detoxification.

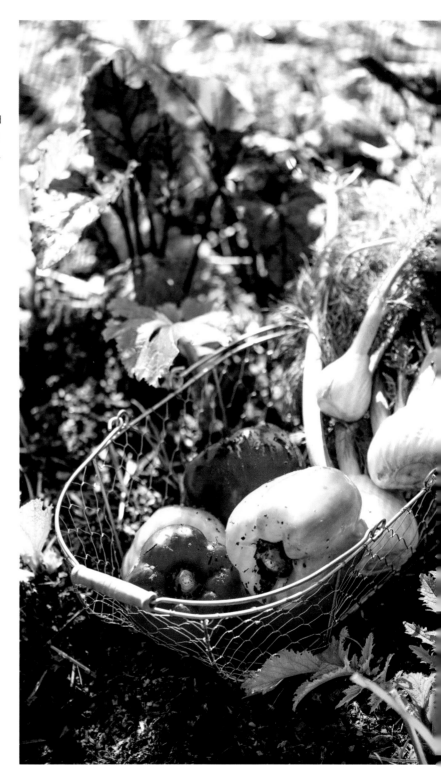

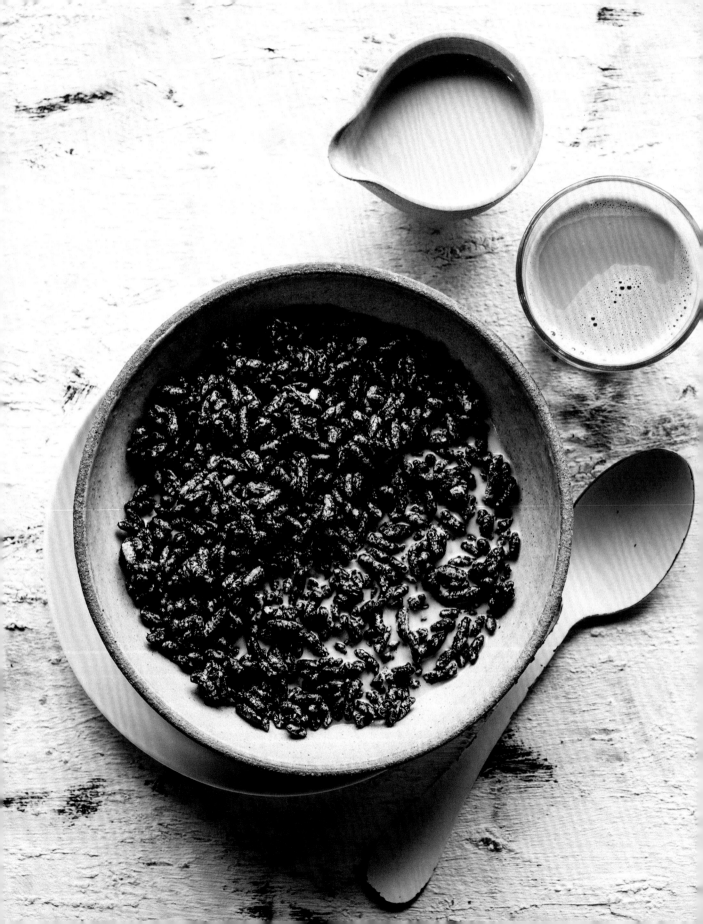

FOR THE WIN: BREAKFAST OF CHAMPIONS

I am quite the morning person and love getting out of bed on the right foot (pun intended), but then I have to kick-start the day with a champion breakfast. These breakfasts are guaranteed to put a smile on your gorgeous face that you'll wear all day. You're welcome!

HOMEMADE CHOCOLATE PUFFED RICE

4 cups puffed brown rice
4 cups puffed white rice
1 Tbsp caramel essence
1 Tbsp vanilla essence
¼ cup almond butter
2 Tbsp olive oil
¼ cup raw honey
3 heaped Tbsp raw cacao powder
2 tsp Oryx desert salt

Preheat the oven to 150 °C and line a baking tray with baking paper.
Mix the brown and white puffed rice in a large mixing bowl.
Combine the remaining ingredients in a small mixing bowl until the almond butter is properly mixed with the olive oil and honey.
Pour over the puffed rice and mix well.
Transfer the mixture to the lined baking tray.
Bake for 8 minutes, then give it a stir and bake for another 7 minutes.
Allow to cool properly for about 45 minutes and then store in an airtight container. It will keep for 1–2 weeks in the pantry or can be frozen for up to 3 months.

NOTE: *One can use 8 cups of either white or brown rice, but I prefer it 50/50. White for the crunch and brown for the fibre.*

SERVINGS: 8–10

All-time favourite! I prefer serving it with unsweetened almond milk and a pinch of love. Now you can enjoy it guilt-free with a healthy smile on your face xxx

BANOFFEE FRENCH TOAST

1 tsp olive oil

3 eggs

½ tsp Oryx desert salt

1 tsp caramel essence

1 tsp raw cacao powder (optional)

2 slices bread of your choice (I prefer 100% rye)

SALTED CARAMEL AND DATE SAUCE

1 cup unsweetened almond milk

300 g fresh pitted Medjool dates

1 cup water

2 tsp caramel essence

1 tsp vanilla essence

1 tsp Oryx desert salt

¼ tsp ground cinnamon

¼ tsp ground nutmeg

1 heaped tsp almond butter

TOPPINGS

almond butter

sliced banana

raw honey

toasted flaked almonds

ground cinnamon

1. First make the sauce. Spray a large saucepan with non-stick cooking spray. Add the almond milk, dates, water, caramel essence, vanilla essence, salt, cinnamon and nutmeg. Cook for 10–15 minutes or until the dates are soft and most of the water has evaporated. Remove from the heat and mash the dates to a smooth consistency. Stir in the almond butter and allow to cool slightly.

2. While the sauce cools, spray a frying pan with non-stick cooking spray and heat the olive oil.

3. In a mixing bowl, beat the eggs, salt and caramel essence until fluffy. If you want to make chocolate French toast, add the cacao powder to the egg mixture now.

4. Soak the bread in the egg mixture, transfer to the frying pan and cook on both sides until toasted and almost crispy.

5. Butter each French toast slice with almond butter and top with banana, followed by honey, toasted flaked almonds and a dusting of cinnamon. Smother in the salted caramel and date sauce.

6. Store any leftover sauce in the fridge for up to 10 days.

NOTE: *To ensure the almond milk in the sauce doesn't curdle, always heat it up with the other ingredients simultaneously.*

SERVINGS: 1

Perfect for Sunday-morning breakfast, Mother's Day and Father's Day, of course, oh, and a birthday breakfast in bed – remember to leave the recipe on the fridge door ;-)

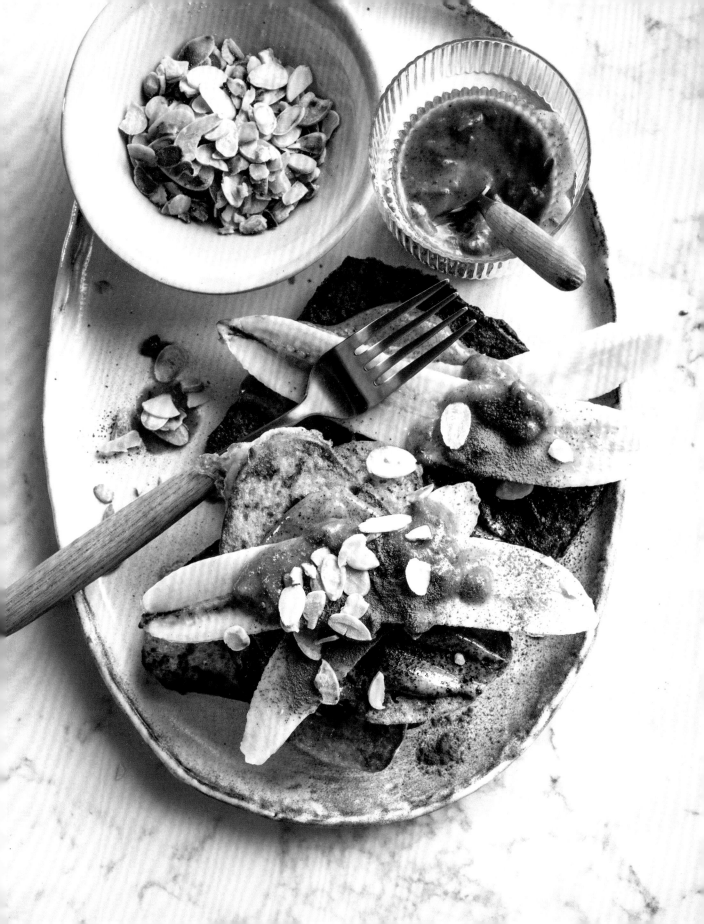

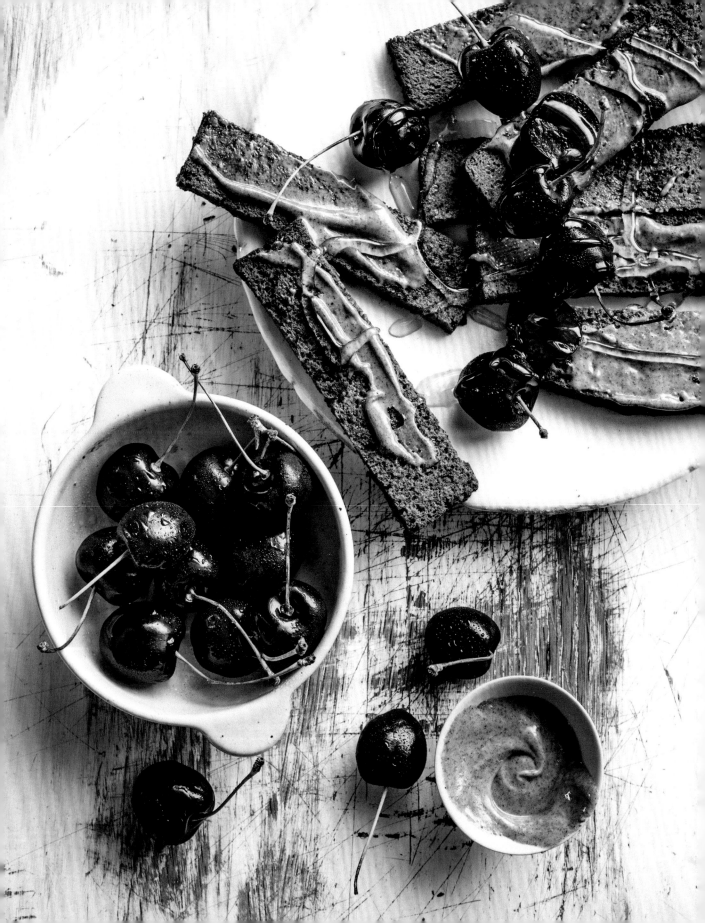

BAKED CINNAMON
FRENCH TOAST STICKS

4 slices bread of your choice (I prefer
100% rye)
2 large eggs
¾ cup unsweetened almond milk
½ tsp ground cinnamon
1 Tbsp raw honey
1 tsp vanilla essence
1 tsp caramel essence
pinch of Oryx desert salt
1 Tbsp olive oil

TOPPINGS
raw honey
almond butter
fresh fruit of your choice

Preheat the oven to 180 °C and line a baking tray with baking paper.
Slice the bread into sticks or soldiers, 3 per slice.
In a mixing bowl, beat the eggs, almond milk, cinnamon, honey, vanilla essence, caramel essence and salt.
Soak the bread sticks in the egg mixture, shake off any excess egg and place them on the lined baking tray, making sure they don't touch.
Drizzle with some of the olive oil (I find a little spray bottle works best) and bake for 10–15 minutes, then flip them over, drizzle with more olive oil and bake for another 10–15 minutes or until cooked through.
Serve topped with honey, almond butter and fresh fruit of your choice.

NOTE: *This is also particularly delicious topped with banana and apple.*

SERVINGS: 2

Quite the favourite as a little spoil in the school lunchbox for first break, just don't forget the I LOVE YOU note! :-)

A lunchbox to work will do the trick as well – even your own :-D

Everyone loves flapjacks!

CHOCOLATE FLAXSEED FLAPJACKS

8 large egg whites (alternatively you
can use 4 whole large eggs)
2 heaped Tbsp ground flaxseeds
1 heaped Tbsp almond flour
1 heaped Tbsp raw cacao powder
1 tsp moringa powder (optional)
1 tsp caramel essence
1 tsp vanilla essence
pinch of Oryx desert salt
1 Tbsp raw honey

TOPPINGS
almond butter
sliced banana
raw honey
flaked almonds
raw cacao powder

1. Place all the ingredients in a mixing bowl and beat to a smooth batter. Alternatively, use a shaker with a whisk ball and shake well for 1 minute.
2. Spray a crêpe pan or small frying pan with non-stick cooking spray and place over medium heat.
3. Pour the batter into the pan, using a quarter of the mixture per flapjack. Cook until bubbles form on the surface, then flip over and cook the other side until golden brown.
4. Top the flapjacks with almond butter, followed by banana, honey, flaked almonds and a dusting of cacao powder.

NOTE: *Lightly toast the flaked almonds for a 'wow' end result!*

SERVINGS: 4 LARGE FLAPJACKS

Top with fresh blueberries instead of banana for another delicious variation

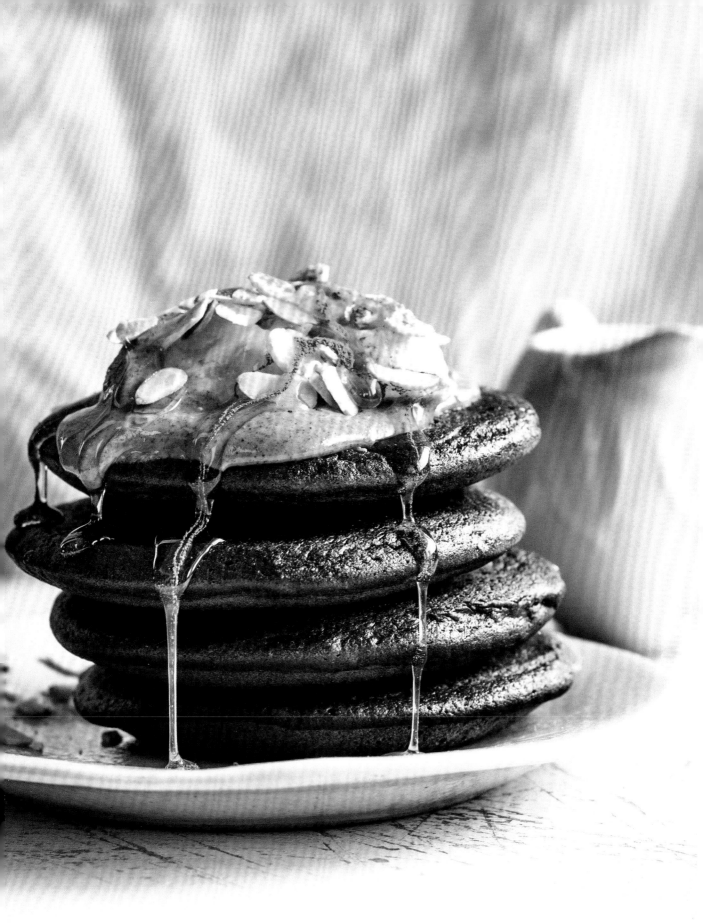

ROOIBOS AND PEAR OATS

1 cup freshly brewed vanilla-flavoured rooibos tea
1 cup unsweetened almond milk
1 cup gluten-free rolled oats
1 x 410 g can unsweetened pear halves, drained and rinsed
½ tsp Oryx desert salt
½ tsp ground cinnamon
1 heaped tsp almond butter
1 Tbsp vanilla essence
1 Tbsp caramel essence
1 Tbsp raw honey
fresh mint for garnishing (optional)

1. Allow the rooibos tea to brew for about 10 minutes while cooling off.
2. Heat the almond milk in a large saucepan over medium heat to about the same temperature as the tea. Add the tea to the milk and then stir in the oats.
3. Add the pears, salt, cinnamon, almond butter, vanilla essence, caramel essence and honey, and simmer for 10–15 minutes or until the mixture starts to thicken.
4. Garnish with fresh mint if desired and serve immediately while lovely and warm.

NOTE: *If vanilla-flavoured rooibos is unavailable, you may use plain rooibos, although the vanilla does add a certain 'wow' factor – a drop of vanilla essence can solve that problem for you.*

SERVINGS: 2

A must try if you're a fan of cooked oats!

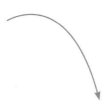

Breakfast on the go!

APPLE CRUMBLE OVERNIGHT OATS

1 cup gluten-free rolled oats
2 cups unsweetened almond milk
1 Tbsp melted almond butter
1 Tbsp raw honey
½ tsp Oryx desert salt
½ tsp ground cinnamon
2 tsp caramel essence

TOPPINGS
sliced fresh apple
raisins
ground cinnamon
toasted flaked almonds
raw honey

In a mixing bowl, combine all the ingredients and refrigerate overnight to set.
Serve the next day topped with apple, raisins, cinnamon, toasted flaked almonds and a drizzle of honey.

NOTE: *Replace the apple slices with fresh blueberries or strawberries for another variation.*

SERVINGS: 2

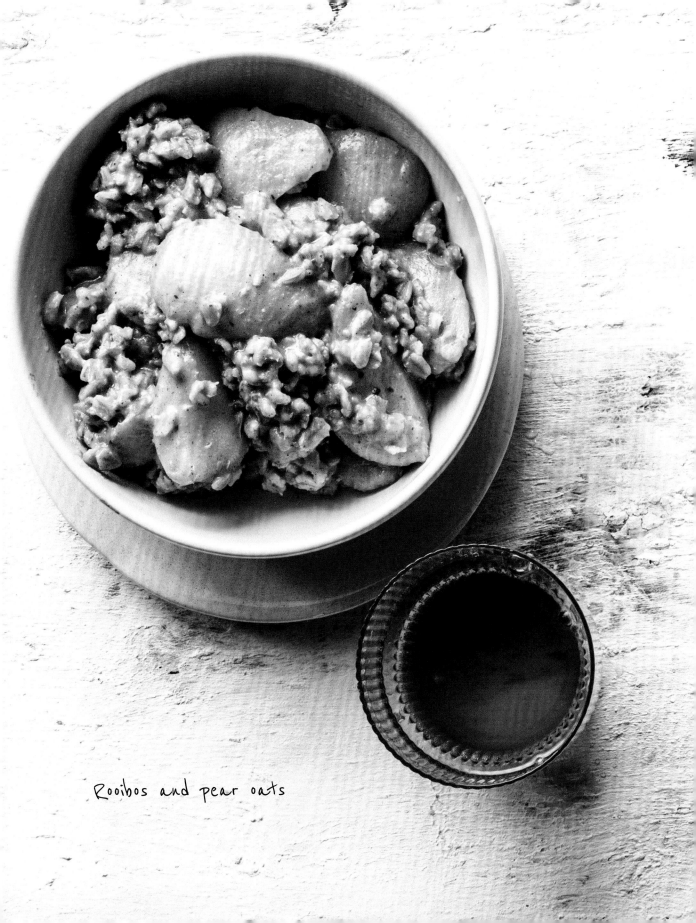

Rooibos and pear oats

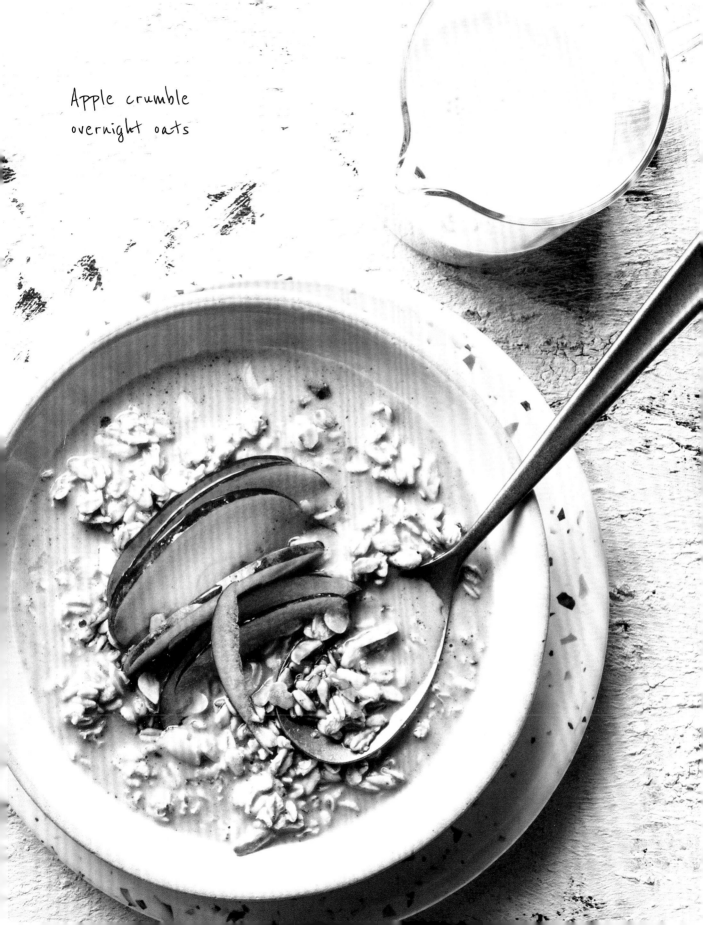

Apple crumble
overnight oats

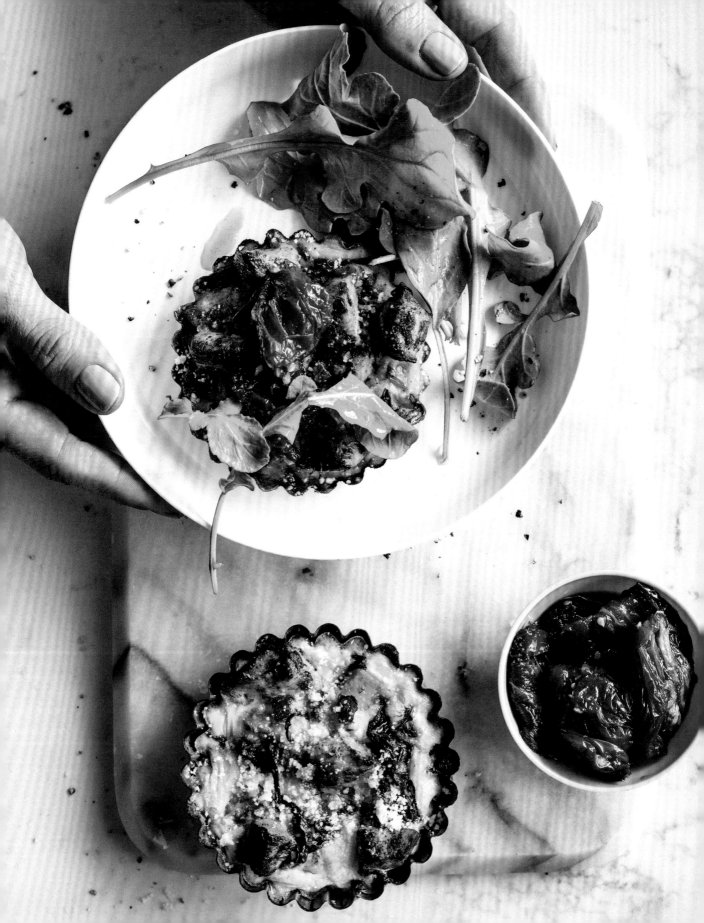

In LOVE with this one!

SMOKY CHICKEN AND BUTTERNUT MINI BREAKFAST QUICHES

CRUST

180 g almond flour, plus extra for dusting
4 tsp raw honey
2 tsp water
¾ tsp Oryx desert salt
¼ tsp ground black pepper, plus extra for garnishing
1 tsp dried parsley

FILLING

50 g baby spinach
200 g butternut, peeled and diced
olive oil
1 medium red onion, finely chopped
2 chicken fillets, diced
1 Tbsp raw honey
1 tsp smoked paprika
1 tsp dried parsley
½ tsp Oryx desert salt
9 eggs

Preheat the oven to 180 °C and spray 6 mini quiche pans with non-stick cooking spray.

Prepare the crust by combining all the ingredients in a mixing bowl.

Scoop 2 heaped Tbsp into each quiche pan, distribute evenly and press down firmly to form a dense crust. Set aside.

Wilt the spinach until soft in boiling water. Drain well and squeeze out all the water.

On the stove or in the microwave, steam the butternut until soft.

Heat a little olive oil in a frying pan and brown the onion. Add the chicken and fry until all the meat is white. Add the honey, paprika, parsley and salt and mix well.

Divide the spinach and butternut between the quiche pans and then top with the chicken mixture.

Whisk the eggs until fluffy and pour over the quiches, filling the pans.

Bake for 20 minutes.

Remove from the oven, drizzle with olive oil and allow to cool before removing the quiches from the pans. Dust each with a little almond flour and finish off with a crack of black pepper.

NOTE: *To make 1 large quiche, use a 23 cm quiche pan or pie dish and bake for 20–25 minutes.*

SERVINGS: 6 MINI QUICHES

Add sundried tomatoes for a tangy twist!

Lunchbox ✓
Roadtripping ✓
Breakfast on the go ✓
Light lunch with salad ✓

QUINOA AND CHICKPEA HASH BROWNS

1 cup cooked quinoa
1 x 410 g can chickpeas, drained, rinsed and pulped
1 small red onion, diced
1 tsp dried parsley
1 tsp chopped fresh ginger
I tsp crushed garlic
1 tsp Oryx desert salt
½ tsp ground black pepper
¼ tsp chilli flakes (optional)
2 Tbsp raw honey
handful of chopped fresh coriander
2 eggs, whisked
1–2 Tbsp almond flour
2 Tbsp olive oil
poached eggs, avocado, lemon cheeks and fresh rocket for serving

Combine the cooked quinoa, chickpeas, onion, parsley, ginger, garlic, salt, pepper, chilli flakes (if using), honey and coriander in a mixing bowl.

Add the whisked eggs and mix well, then add the almond flour until you reach a firm consistency.

Using your hands, form the mixture into 6–8 hash browns of whatever size you prefer.

Heat the olive oil in a frying pan and cook the hash browns on both sides until brown and crisp – about 10 minutes. Be careful, as they will only start firming up properly once cooked and cooled.

Serve with poached eggs, avocado, lemon cheeks and fresh rocket.

NOTE: *Spray your hands with non-stick cooking spray or use a drop of olive oil to ensure the mixture doesn't stick to your hands when forming the hash browns.*

SERVINGS: 6–8 HASH BROWNS

You can use these hash browns as vegetarian burger patties too

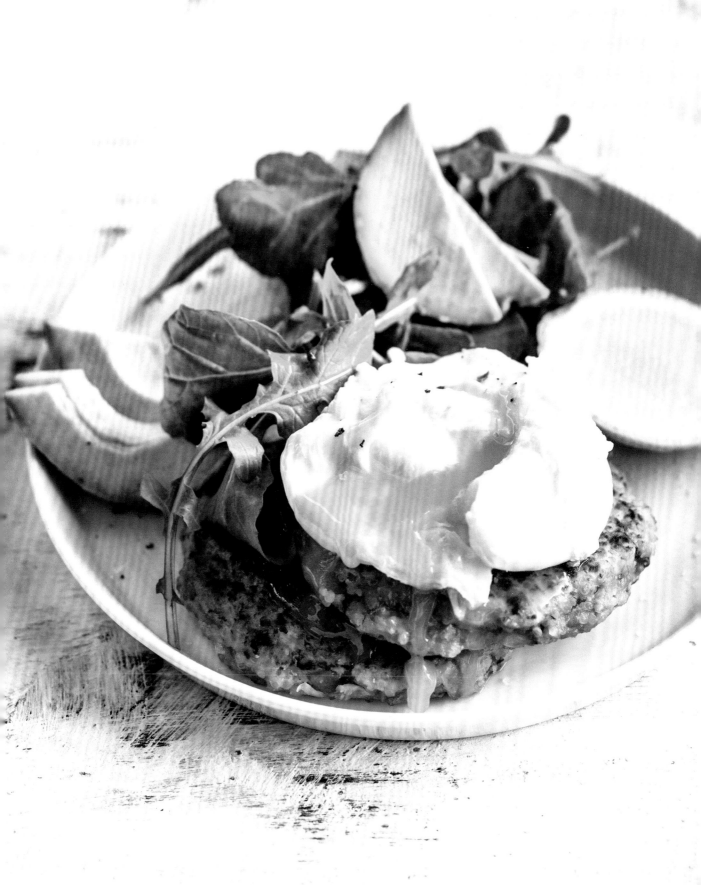

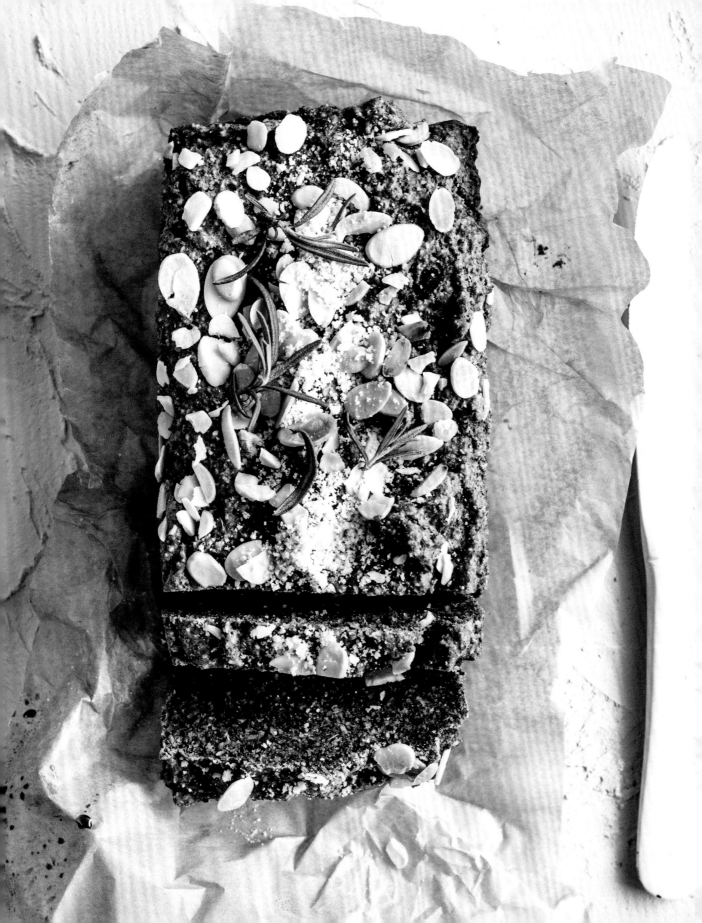

ROSEMARY ALMOND BREAD

1½ cups almond flour, plus extra
for dusting
4 heaped Tbsp flaxseed flour
1 tsp dried thyme
½ tsp Oryx desert salt
¼ tsp ground black pepper
1 Tbsp bicarbonate of soda
2 Tbsp chopped fresh rosemary
1 Tbsp apple cider vinegar
¼ cup olive oil
5 large eggs, whisked
1 Tbsp flaked almonds

Preheat the oven to 180 °C and line a standard loaf pan with baking paper.

Mix the almond flour, flaxseed flour, thyme, salt, black pepper, bicarbonate of soda and rosemary in a mixing bowl, then add the apple cider vinegar and olive oil. Add the whisked eggs and mix until well blended.

Pour the batter into the lined loaf pan (don't fill it more than three-quarters full), dust with almond flour and sprinkle the flaked almonds evenly on top.

Bake for 30 minutes. Allow to cool slightly in the pan before turning out and serving.

NOTE: *Make sure you mix all the dry ingredients well to incorporate the bicarbonate of soda evenly.*

SERVINGS: 1 LOAF

Dad's FAVOURITE!!! Perfect to bake any time, but especially on Father's Day!

OVEN-ROASTED PAPAYA WITH BANANA AND PECAN NUTS

2 medium papayas, halved
and deseeded
2 bananas, mashed
1 heaped Tbsp almond flour
½ tsp Oryx desert salt
2 tsp caramel essence
½ tsp ground cinnamon
2 Tbsp raw honey
50 g pecan nuts, chopped

TOPPINGS
crushed Ryvita
chia seeds
chopped pecan nuts
raw honey
almond flour
chopped fresh thyme
lime juice

1. Preheat the oven to 200 °C and spray a baking tray with non-stick cooking spray.
2. Place the papaya halves, cut-side up, on the greased tray.
3. In a bowl, mix the mashed bananas with the rest of the ingredients and use this mixture to fill the papaya halves.
4. Top with as much crushed Ryvita, chia seeds and pecan nuts as you like, drizzle with honey and roast for 15–20 minutes or until the filling is golden and the nuts toasted.
5. Serve garnished with a sprinkle of almond flour, fresh thyme and a squeeze of lime juice.

SERVINGS: 4

A must try if you're a fan of papaya & banana

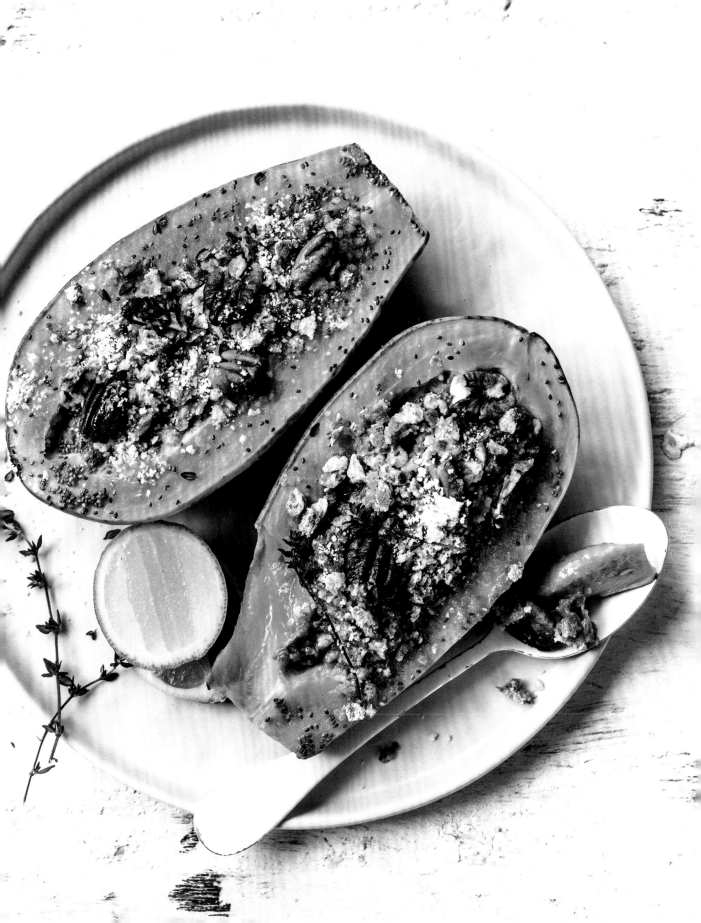

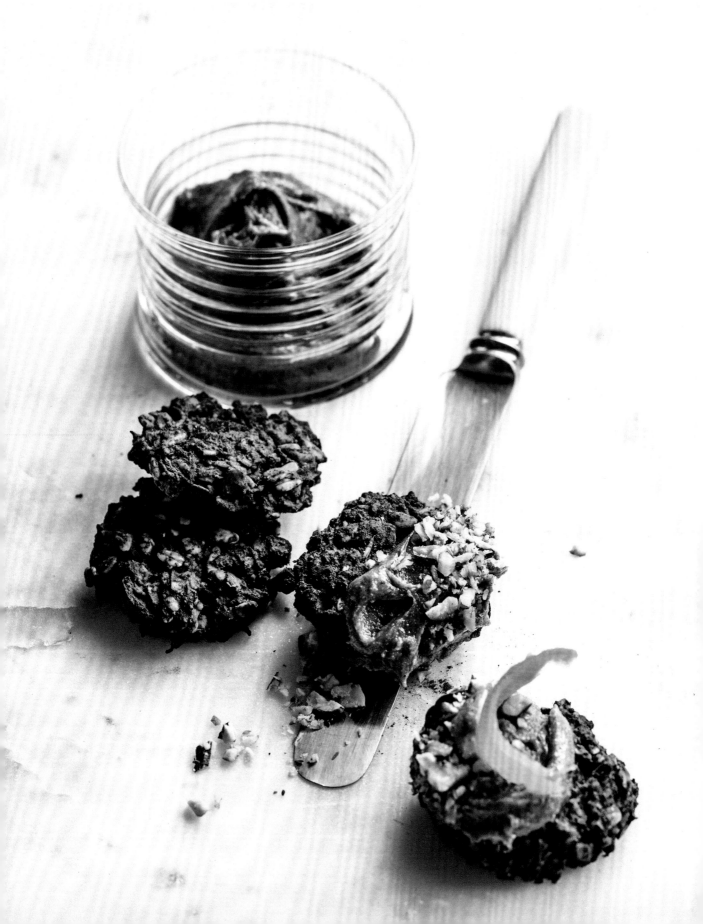

It's like carrot cake for busy people :-P

CARROT CAKE BREAKFAST BISCUITS

¾ cup unsweetened almond milk
½ cup almond butter
1 tsp vanilla essence
1 tsp caramel essence
1 medium banana, mashed
6 Tbsp raw honey
1 cup finely grated carrot
2 Tbsp ground flaxseeds
1 tsp bicarbonate of soda
1 tsp Oryx desert salt
2 tsp ground cinnamon
1½ cups gluten-free rolled oats
½ cup almond flour, plus extra for dusting
100 g pecan nuts, chopped, plus extra for garnishing
100 g pitted dates, chopped

ICING

180 g almond butter
1¼ tsp Oryx desert salt
¼ cup raw honey
2 tsp caramel essence
1 tsp ground cinnamon

Preheat the oven to 180 °C and line a baking tray with baking paper.

In a large mixing bowl, mix the almond milk, almond butter, vanilla essence, caramel essence, banana, honey, carrot and flaxseeds.

Stir in the rest of the ingredients.

Roll the mixture into small balls and place them on the lined tray. Using a fork dipped in ground cinnamon, gently flatten the balls.

Bake for 25 minutes. Allow to cool completely before icing.

To make the icing, mix all the ingredients in a small bowl. Spread over the cooled biscuits, dust with almond flour and garnish with extra chopped pecan nuts.

Store in an airtight container in the fridge.

SERVINGS: 25–30 BISCUITS

Who said you can't have cake before breakfast?!!!

100% Mom-approved :-D

The perfect way to sneak vegetables into breakfast ... disguised as a chocolate smoothie

ROAST SWEET POTATO AND CHOCOLATE BREAKFAST SMOOTHIE

3 egg whites
150 ml unsweetened almond milk
pinch of Oryx desert salt
1 tsp caramel essence
1 heaped tsp raw cacao powder
1 tsp almond butter
100 g frozen oven-roasted sweet potatoes (see page 43)
2 tsp raw honey
1 tsp olive oil
¼ tsp ground cinnamon (optional)
flaked almonds and fresh mint or thyme for garnishing

1. Place all the ingredients, except the garnish, in a blender and blend until smooth.
2. Serve immediately, garnished with flaked almonds and fresh mint or thyme.

SERVINGS: 1 LARGE OR 2 MEDIUM SMOOTHIES

Frozen sweet potato can be added to any flavour smoothie for a creamy, low-GI, anti-inflammatory boost!

#you'rewelcome

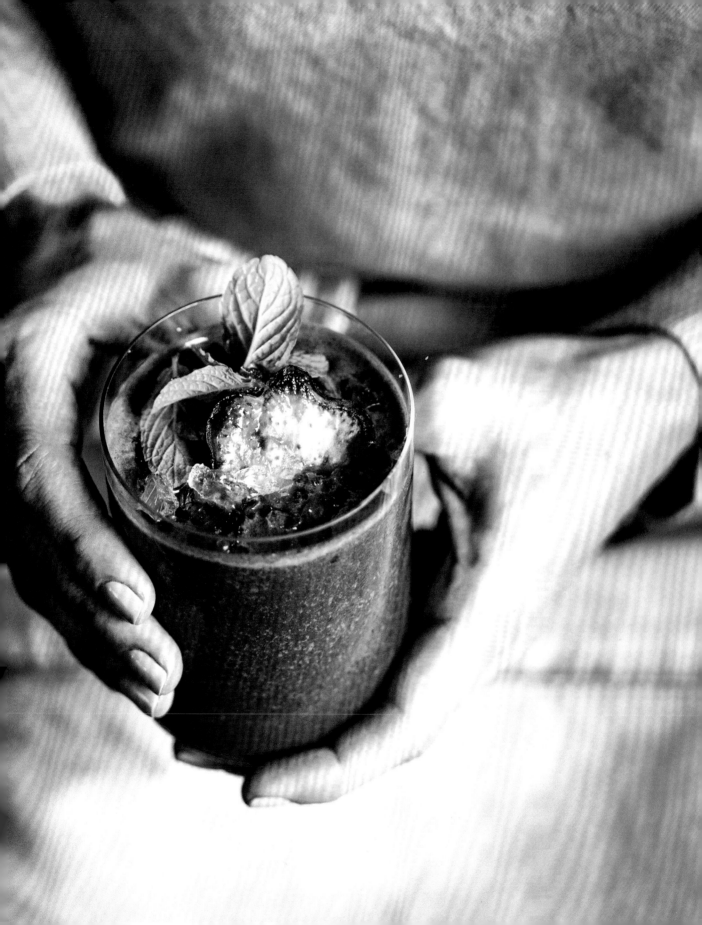

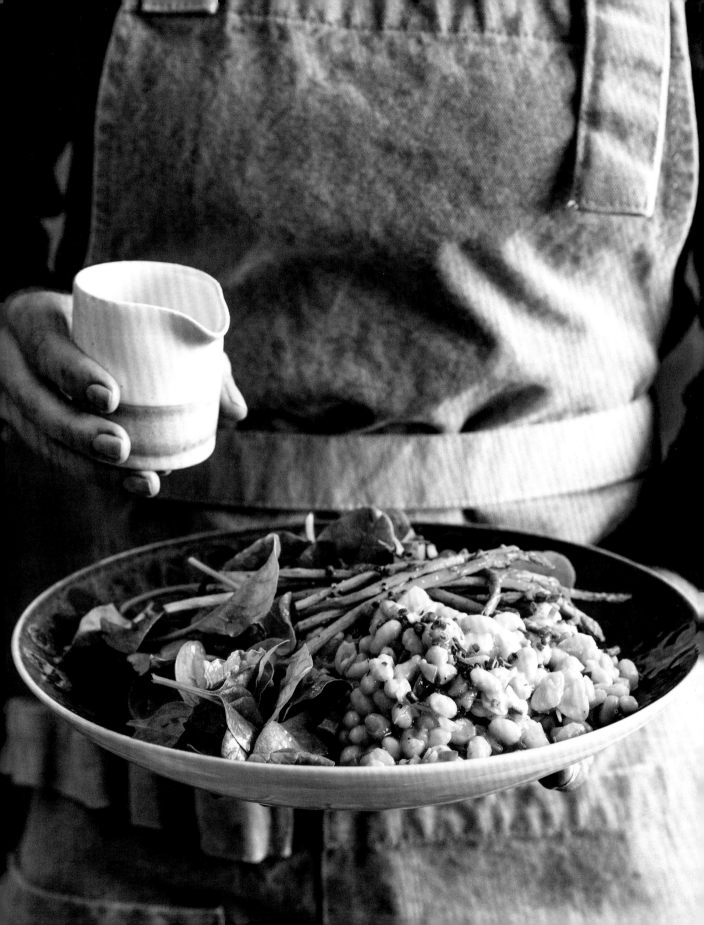

MOTIVATION MONDAY

New week, new opportunities to be the best version of yourself! But are you ready for the busy week ahead with regards to meals? Here is my go-to meal-prep guide. I always try to have base meals in the fridge, because, let's be honest, convenience is key.

Replace with long-stem broccoli if you're not a fan of asparagus

CANNELLINI BEAN SALAD WITH CARAMEL CHILLI-LIME DRESSING

100 g whole young asparagus
olive oil
Oryx desert salt
ground black pepper
1 red onion, diced
1 pimiento or red bell pepper, deseeded and diced
1 heaped tsp crushed garlic
50 g flaked almonds
2 x 400 g cans cannellini beans, drained and rinsed
100 g baby spinach

CARAMEL CHILLI-LIME DRESSING

juice of 2 limes
1 tsp caramel essence
¼ tsp chilli flakes
1 tsp dried parsley
1 tsp Oryx desert salt
¼ tsp ground black pepper
3 Tbsp raw honey
3 Tbsp olive oil
5–6 Tbsp chopped fresh chives

Preheat the oven to 200 °C and spray a baking tray with non-stick cooking spray.

Place the asparagus on the tray, drizzle with olive oil and season with salt and black pepper. Roast for about 15 minutes or until cooked to preference. Set aside to cool.

Heat a drizzle of olive oil in a frying pan over medium heat and fry the onion, pimiento or red bell pepper, garlic and flaked almonds until the vegetables are soft and the almonds are toasted.

Remove from the heat and allow to cool slightly before adding to the cannellini beans in a large bowl. Be careful not to stir too much, as it will ruin the appearance of the beans. Add the whole grilled asparagus.

Mix all the dressing ingredients in a jug and pour over the bean salad.

Refrigerate for at least 1 hour to allow the salad to chill properly.

Serve with the baby spinach and enjoy as a main meal or side.

NOTE: *This is the ideal salad to pair with a protein of your choice. It also works wonders with quinoa and even basmati or brown rice.*

SERVINGS: 4

No cannellini? No problem! Replace with either butterbeans or chickpeas

HONEY-MUSTARD AND ROSEMARY CHICKEN TRAY BAKE

1.5 kg chicken fillets
brine (3 Tbsp Oryx desert salt
dissolved in 1.2 litres water)
2 Tbsp olive oil
2 Tbsp raw honey
1 Tbsp onion powder
1 Tbsp mustard powder
1 Tbsp mustard seeds
1 Tbsp dried rosemary
½ tsp ground black pepper
½ tsp Oryx desert salt

1. Soak the chicken fillets overnight in the brine.
2. When ready to cook, preheat the oven to 180 °C. Line a roasting tray with baking paper or foil and spray with non-stick cooking spray if you want to make your life easier and skip the scrubbing afterwards.
3. Remove the chicken from the brine and pat dry with paper towel.
4. Arrange the chicken fillets on the tray and drizzle first with the olive oil and then with the honey. Sprinkle over the onion powder, followed by the mustard powder, mustard seeds and dried rosemary respectively, in this order. Finish off with the black pepper.
5. Bake in the oven for 25 minutes.
6. Remove from the oven and drain the juices (if you would like to make a sauce, pour these juices into a saucepan with some of the ingredients used in the recipe and simmer until thickened).
7. Sprinkle the salt over the chicken and allow to cool properly before placing in an airtight container and storing in the fridge to use when needed.

NOTE: *The trick for the most tender oven-baked chicken is to soak the fillets overnight in brine before baking and to only season with salt once the chicken is cooked.*

SERVINGS: 10

Both of these chicken tray bakes are great with salad, sweet potato, butternut, roast vegetables and even brown or basmati rice

SWEET BASIL
BBQ CHICKEN TRAY BAKE

1.5 kg chicken fillets
brine (3 Tbsp Oryx desert salt
dissolved in 1.2 litres water)
2 Tbsp olive oil
2 Tbsp raw honey
1 Tbsp paprika
1 Tbsp dried sweet basil
1 Tbsp onion flakes
½ tsp ground black pepper
½ tsp Oryx desert salt

Soak the chicken fillets overnight in the brine.

When ready to cook, preheat the oven to 180 °C. Line a roasting tray with baking paper or foil and spray with non-stick cooking spray.

Remove the chicken from the brine and pat dry with paper towel.

Arrange the chicken fillets on the tray and drizzle first with the olive oil and then with the honey. Sprinkle with the paprika, sweet basil and onion flakes respectively, in this order. Finish off with the black pepper.

Bake in the oven for 25 minutes.

Remove from the oven and drain the juices (if you would like to make a sauce, pour these juices into a saucepan with some of the ingredients used in the recipe and simmer until thickened).

Sprinkle the salt over the chicken and allow to cool properly before placing in an airtight container and storing in the fridge to use when needed.

SERVINGS: 10

OVEN-ROASTED SWEET POTATOES

1 kg sweet potatoes, washed not scrubbed, otherwise you'll remove the skin which contains most of the fibre

Preheat the oven to 200 °C. Line a baking tray with foil and spray with non-stick cooking spray.

Soak the whole sweet potatoes in water for 5–10 minutes.

Cut off the ends and roughly cut the sweet potatoes into chunks.

Place the sweet potato chunks on the lined baking tray and bake for 1 hour 15 minutes.

Allow to cool before placing in an airtight container and storing in the fridge to use when needed. They will last up to 5 days refrigerated. Also freeze some to add to smoothies (see page 38). If serving on the same day as roasting, drizzle with olive oil and raw honey and season with salt.

SERVINGS: 4–5

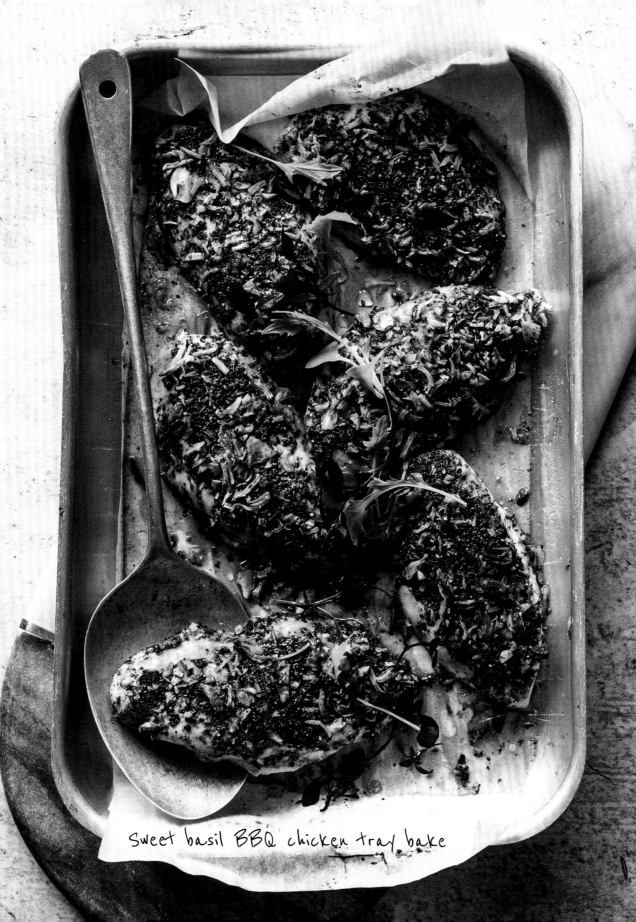

Sweet basil BBQ chicken tray bake

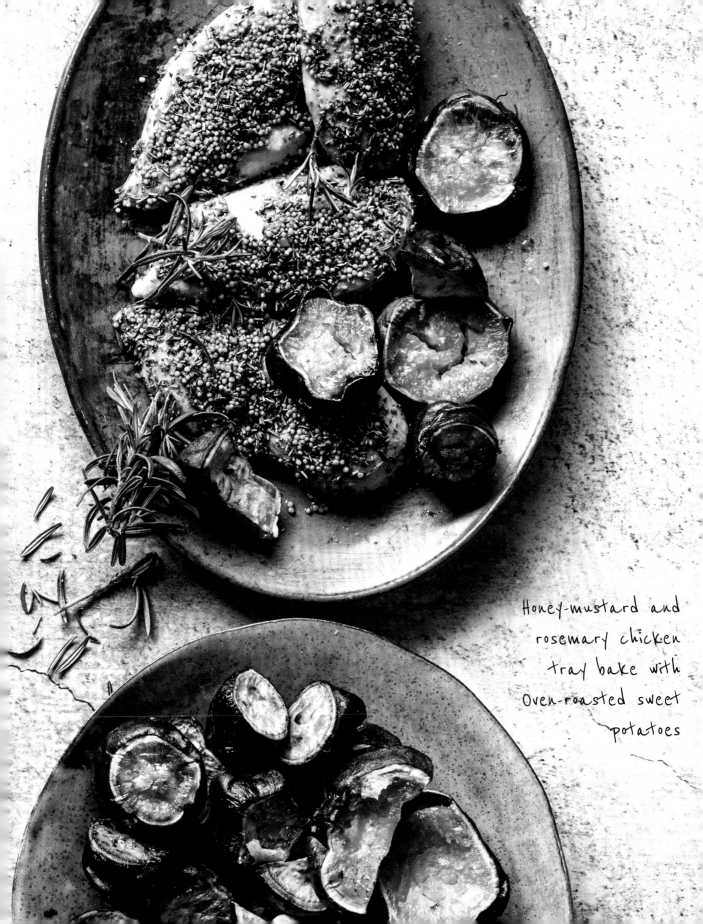

Honey-mustard and rosemary chicken tray bake with oven-roasted sweet potatoes

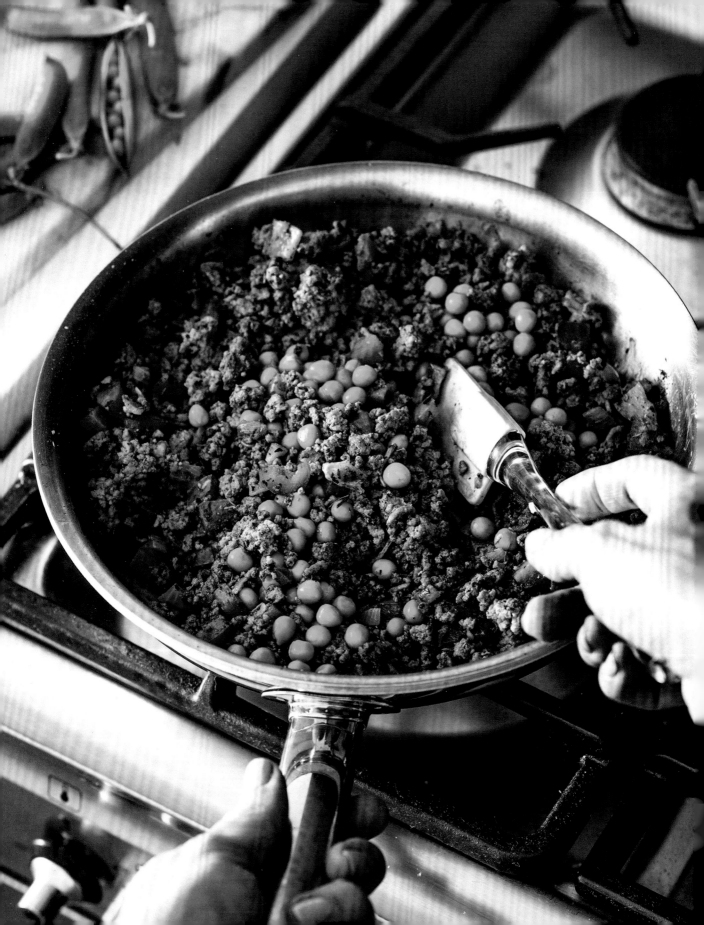

Perfect to pair with vegetables and/or rice

PIQUANTÉ PEPPER, BASIL, PEA AND THYME MINCE

1 Tbsp olive oil
2 red onions, diced
1.5 kg extra-lean mince
120 g Piquanté Peppers, chopped
4 tsp Oryx desert salt
1 tsp ground black pepper
¼ cup raw honey
3 heaped Tbsp paprika
1 heaped Tbsp dried sweet basil
2 heaped tsp dried thyme
4 heaped tsp onion flakes
250 g frozen peas, defrosted

Heat the olive oil in a large frying pan and brown the onions.

Add the mince and cook for about 15 minutes until most of the liquid has evaporated and the mince is pale brown.

Add the Piquanté Peppers, salt, black pepper, honey, paprika, sweet basil, thyme and onion flakes and stir well.

Lastly, add the defrosted peas and simmer for another 5–10 minutes.

Allow to cool before placing in an airtight container and storing in the fridge to use when needed.

NOTE: *This makes an amazing base for a sweet potato cottage pie.*

SERVINGS: 8–10

QUICK AND EASY HEAVENLY HAKE FILLETS

800 g frozen hake fillets
1 tsp Oryx desert salt
1 tsp paprika
½ tsp harissa powder or pinch of
chilli flakes
1 tsp dried parsley
1 red onion, diced
1 Tbsp olive oil
chopped fresh parsley for garnishing

1. Preheat the oven to 200 °C and spray a roasting tray with non-stick cooking spray.
2. Place the frozen hake fillets on the tray and bake for 10 minutes.
3. Remove from the oven and sprinkle the fish first with the salt, then with the paprika, harissa or chilli flakes and parsley respectively.
4. Scatter the onion over the hake fillets and return to the oven for another 10 minutes.
5. Remove from the oven, drizzle with the olive oil and then bake for another 10 minutes until golden brown and crispy.
6. Serve garnished with chopped fresh parsley. The fish can be stored in the fridge for up to 2 days.

NOTE: *You may also use fresh hake fillets. If you do, skip step 2.*

SERVINGS: 4

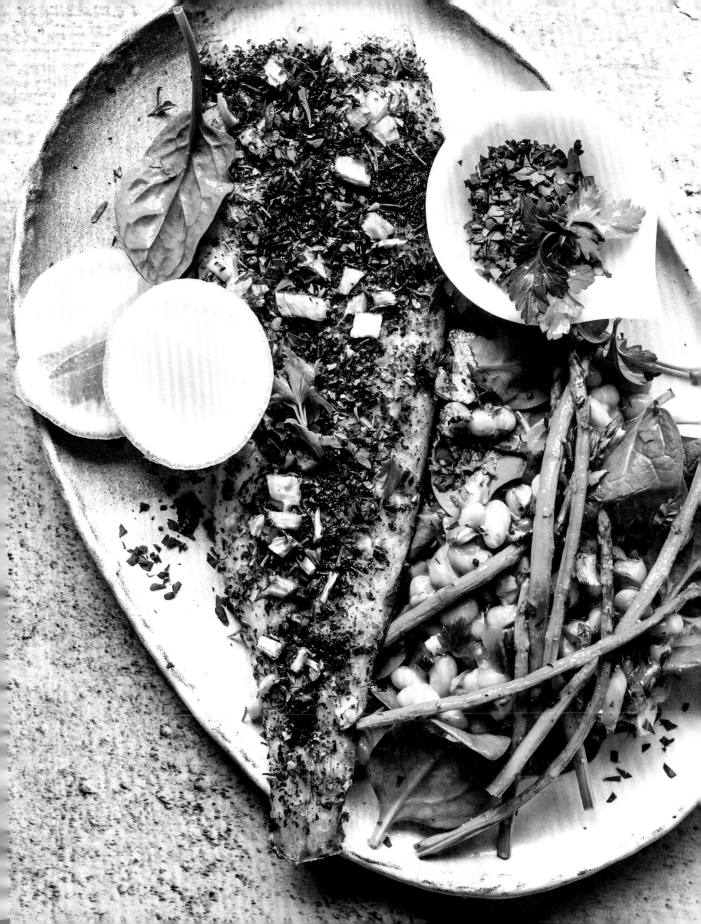

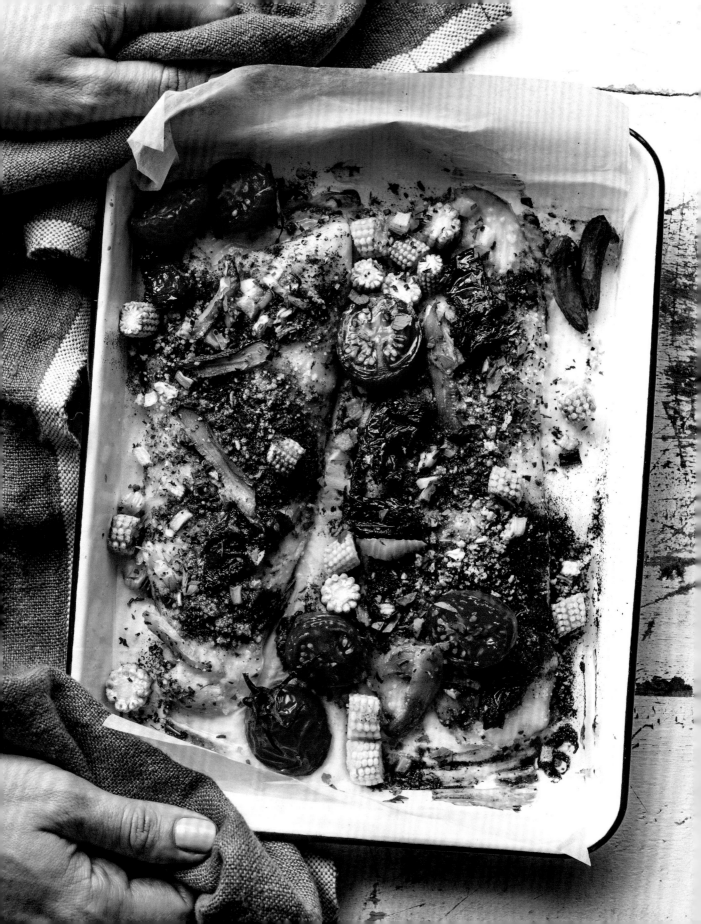

ANTIPASTI-STYLE HAKE FILLETS

800 g frozen hake fillets
½ tsp Oryx desert salt
1 tsp paprika
20 g almond flour
½ tsp harissa powder or pinch of chilli flakes
⅓ white onion, finely diced
4 sweet-and-sour gherkins, cut into thin strips
30 g sundried tomatoes, cut into strips with kitchen scissors
100 g baby corn, cut into chunks
300 g vine tomatoes, halved
1 Tbsp raw honey
1 tsp balsamic vinegar
½ tsp dried sweet basil or dried origanum
handful of pitted black olives (optional)

Preheat the oven to 200 °C and spray a roasting tray with non-stick cooking spray.
Place the frozen hake fillets on the tray and bake for 10 minutes.
Remove from the oven and sprinkle the fish first with the salt, then with the paprika, almond flour, harissa or chilli flakes and onion respectively.
Top the fillets with the gherkins and sundried tomatoes.
Arrange the baby corn and vine tomatoes around the fish on the baking tray and drizzle everything with the honey and balsamic vinegar.
Sprinkle over the sweet basil or origanum and return to the oven for another 20 minutes.
If using, garnish with the olives before serving. The fish can be stored in the fridge for up to 2 days.

NOTE: *You may also use fresh hake fillets. If you do, skip step 2.*

SERVINGS: 4

Perfect for the dinner table, these are a bit more sophisticated for when you have dinner guests

A perfect addition to any snack platter

CHICKEN MEATBALLS

1 kg chicken mince
1 large red onion, diced
1 medium red bell pepper or
2 medium pimiento peppers,
diced (keep the seeds)
1 tsp crushed garlic
2 tsp onion powder
1 Tbsp soy sauce
1 Tbsp raw honey
1 tsp Oryx desert salt
½ tsp ground black pepper
handful of chopped fresh basil
1 large egg, whisked
1 tsp sesame seeds
½ tsp raw honey
½ tsp olive oil

1. Preheat the oven to 200 °C and spray an ovenproof dish with non-stick cooking spray.
2. In a large mixing bowl, combine the chicken mince, onion, bell or pimiento peppers and reserved seeds.
3. Add the garlic, onion powder, soy sauce, 1 Tbsp honey, salt, black pepper and basil. Mix well.
4. Add the egg and mix well.
5. Roll the mixture into balls and place in the greased dish. Sprinkle over the sesame seeds.
6. Bake for 15 minutes, then remove from the oven and drizzle with the ½ tsp honey and olive oil. Return to the oven for another 2–3 minutes.
7. Allow to cool before placing in an airtight container and storing in the fridge to use when needed.

SERVINGS: 16–18 MEATBALLS

Pop in your picnic basket or pack as padkos – these are easy and convenient to eat with your hands :-D

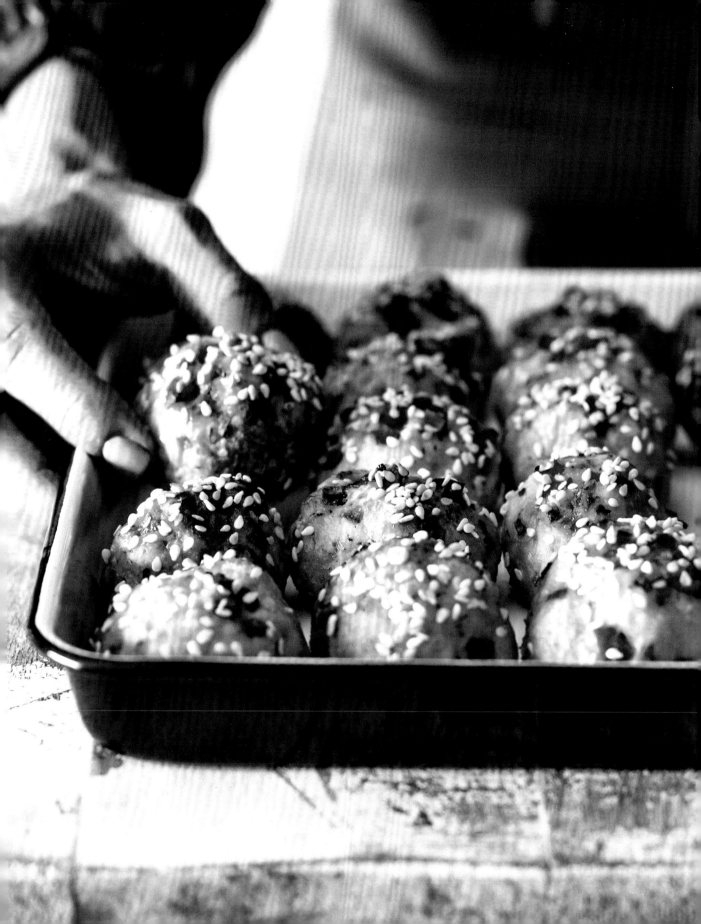

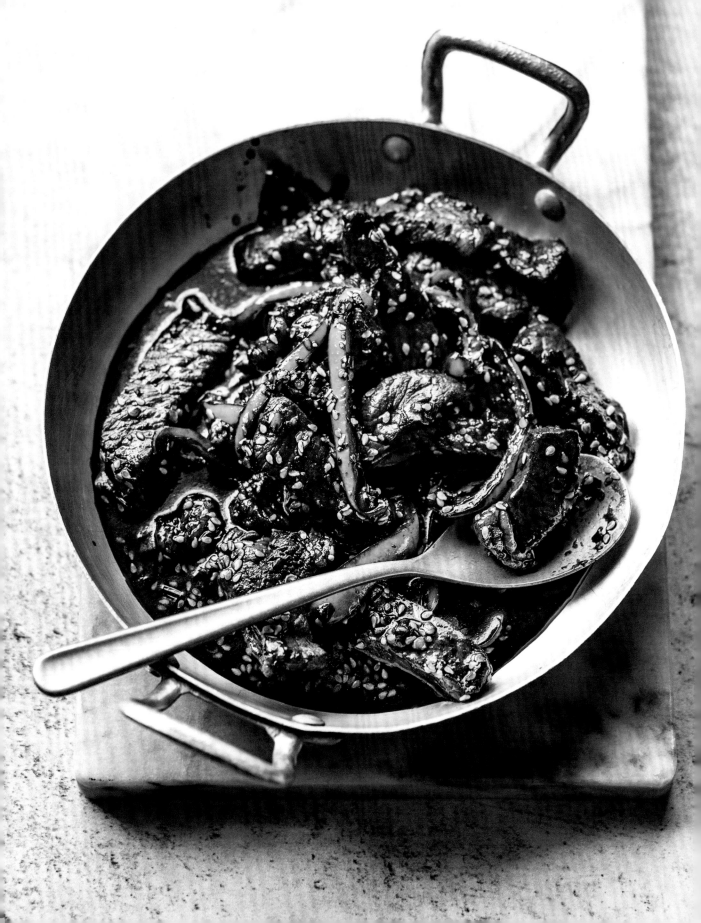

SOY AND SESAME BEEF STRIPS

2 Tbsp olive oil
3 spring onions, chopped
1 heaped tsp crushed garlic
1 medium red, orange or yellow bell
pepper, cut into strips (keep
the seeds)
600 g beef strips
5 Tbsp soy sauce or tamari
2 Tbsp sesame seeds
1 tsp ground black pepper
¼ cup raw honey
½ tsp Oryx desert salt
handful of chopped fresh
Italian parsley

Heat the olive oil in a frying pan over medium heat and fry the spring onions, garlic, bell pepper and reserved seeds for about 5 minutes to release their flavour, then add the beef strips and fry until the meat is golden brown.

In a small bowl, mix the soy sauce or tamari, sesame seeds, black pepper, honey and salt. Add this to the pan once the meat is cooked, and simmer for about 15 minutes or until most of the moisture has evaporated.

Add the chopped fresh parsley, remove from the heat and allow to cool completely before placing in an airtight container and storing in the fridge to use when needed.

NOTE: *Be on the lookout for tamari, a more mature gluten-free alternative to soy sauce.*

SERVINGS: 4

A winner served with rice and green beans!

Something to keep the vegetarians happy :-P

QUINOA WITH TOASTED SEEDS, ROSEMARY AND THYME

1 cup cooked quinoa
1 tsp dried rosemary
1 tsp dried thyme
¼ tsp ground black pepper
1½ tsp Oryx desert salt
2 Tbsp olive oil
1 medium red onion, diced
100 g pumpkin seeds
2 heaped Tbsp sesame seeds
2 Tbsp raw honey
1 heaped Tbsp almond flour
handful of chopped fresh thyme

1. Place the cooked quinoa in a bowl and add the rosemary, thyme, black pepper and ½ tsp of the salt. Set aside.
2. Heat the olive oil in a frying pan and fry the onion until it just starts to brown. Add the pumpkin and sesame seeds and stir continuously until the onion is brown and the seeds start to pop.
3. Add the honey and remaining salt and keep stirring until the honey has caramelised.
4. Add the almond flour and stir until the pumpkin seeds are well coated.
5. Remove from the heat and stir into the quinoa. Sprinkle over the chopped fresh thyme.
6. Allow to cool completely before placing in an airtight container and storing in the fridge to use when needed.

NOTE: *Tasty, easy and versatile, this is an add-any-additional-vegetable, plant-based protein option! Served with oven-roasted vegetables, it's a real show-stopper.*

SERVINGS: 6—8

Add some 'crisp' to the 'crunch' with some leafy greens like baby spinach

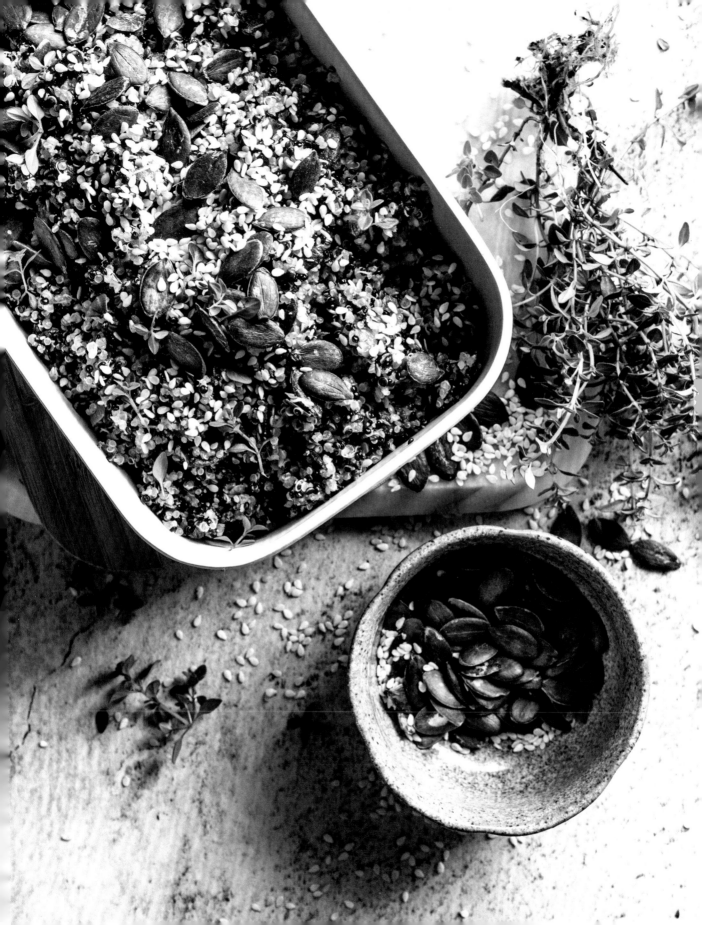

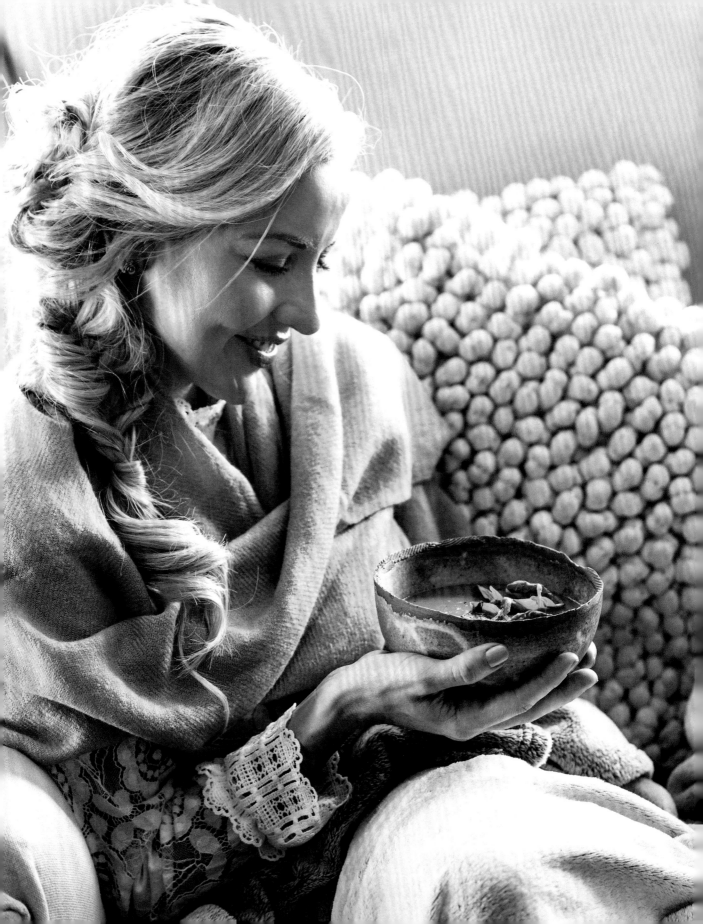

I LOVE ME xoxo ... my favourites

Invite your scarf and slippers, because we're having a slumber party! This chapter is all about sharing a snuggle with a bowl on a cold winter's day. Soups, casseroles and warm puddings ... mmm. Word on the street is that summer bodies are made in winter. This may be true, but if you can work on that summer body while enjoying some winter-warmer goodness, sign me up!

ROSA TOMATO AND BASIL SOUP

1 Tbsp olive oil

1 medium red onion, diced

½ Tbsp crushed garlic

1.5 kg rosa tomatoes, halved

½ cup chopped fresh basil, plus extra for serving

2 tsp dried sweet basil

1 Tbsp Oryx desert salt

1 tsp ground black pepper (optional)

4 heaped tsp paprika

3 Tbsp raw honey

2 Tbsp balsamic vinegar

1 cup unsweetened almond milk

4 cups hot water

thinly sliced moist biltong for serving (optional)

In a large saucepan, heat the olive oil and fry the onion until golden brown. Add the garlic and stir.

Add the rosa tomatoes, fresh basil, dried sweet basil, salt, black pepper (if using), paprika, honey and balsamic vinegar. Simmer for 10 minutes.

Add the almond milk and hot water and simmer for a further 40–45 minutes, stirring occasionally.

Blend to the desired texture and serve garnished with extra fresh basil and thinly sliced moist biltong (if desired).

NOTE: *Serve with freshly baked rosemary almond bread (see page 33) for a complete meal.*

SERVINGS: 6–8

Black pepper helps you absorb nutrients, so add with love to get the most of this easy yet heart-warming soup

Always a crowd-pleaser!

FARM-STYLE BEEF AND VEGETABLE SOUP

1 Tbsp olive oil
1 medium red onion, diced
500 g extra-lean beef mince
½ cup chopped fresh Italian parsley
500 g rosa tomatoes, halved
425 g fresh or defrosted frozen peas
550 g carrots, sliced
300 g spinach, chopped
500 g sweet potatoes, cut into chunks
15 cups (3.75 litres) hot water
1 tsp crushed garlic
¼ cup balsamic vinegar
2 heaped Tbsp paprika
2 Tbsp raw honey
2 tsp Oryx desert salt
1 tsp Oryx desert wine salt
1 tsp ground black pepper
2 tsp garlic flakes
2 tsp dried sweet basil

1. In a large saucepan, heat the olive oil and fry the onion until golden brown. Add the mince and parsley, and fry until the mince is cooked.
2. In the meantime, spray a separate saucepan with non-stick cooking spray and cook the rosa tomatoes for about 10 minutes until soft, then add to the mince.
3. Add the peas, carrots, spinach, sweet potatoes and 11 cups (2.75 litres) of the hot water. Give it a good stir and bring to a light simmer.
4. Add the remaining ingredients, reduce the heat to low and simmer for 30–45 minutes, adding the remaining 4 cups water while it cooks. Stir occasionally and cook until the vegetables are soft and tender.

NOTE: *Serve with freshly baked rosemary almond bread (see page 33) for a complete meal.*

SERVINGS: 10–12

*Inspired by Mom's favourite soup :-)
Ideal for freezing!*

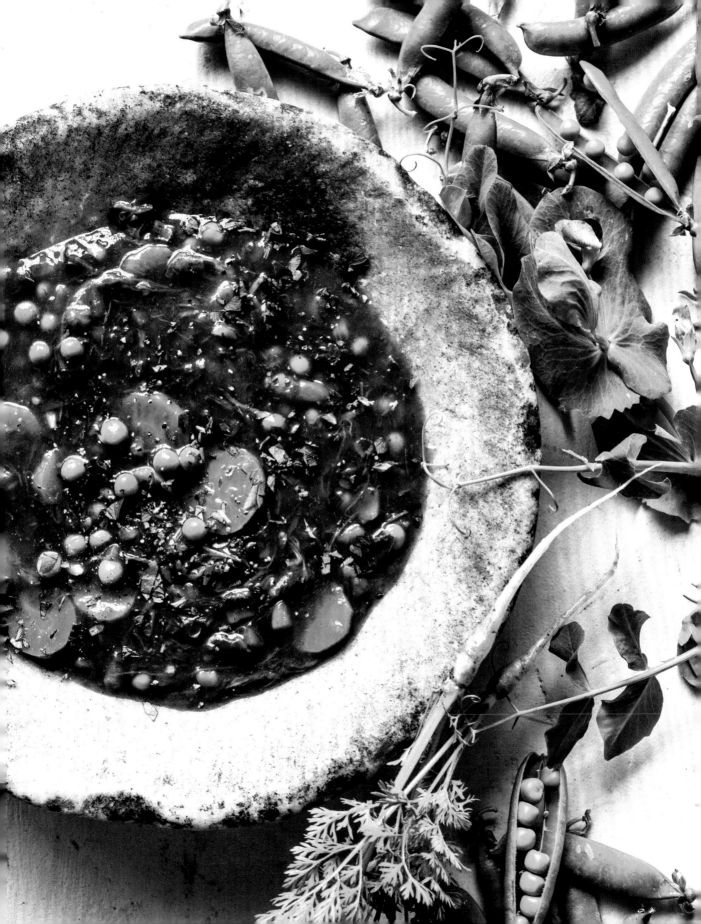

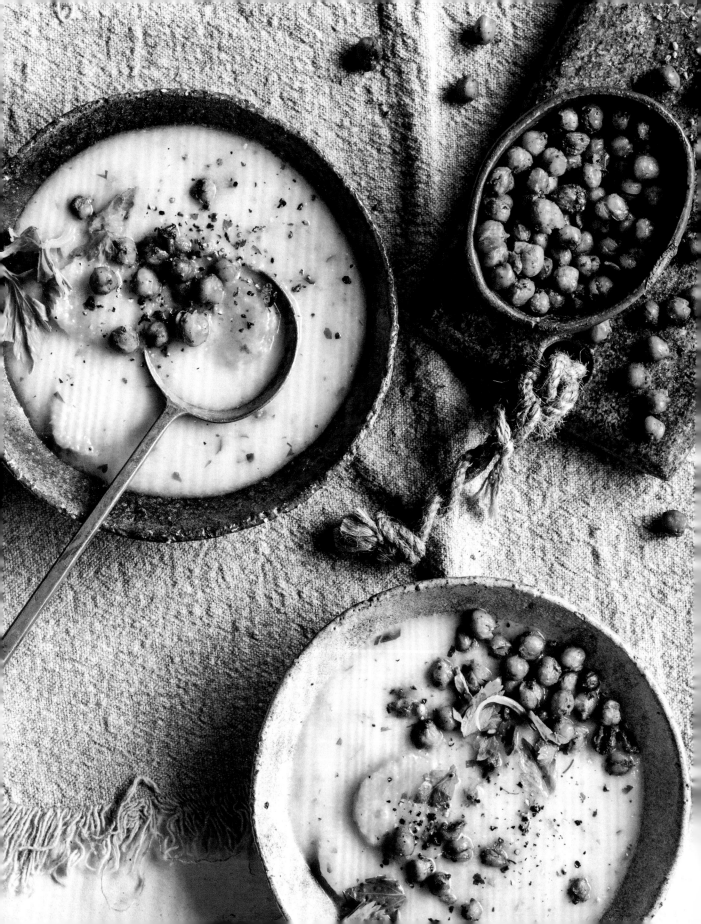

Pretty & perfect when having guests over!

CREAMY GARLIC AND BUTTERBEAN SOUP WITH OVEN-ROASTED CHICKPEAS

2 Tbsp olive oil
4 x 410 g cans butterbeans, drained
and processed or blended
until smooth
8 cups unsweetened almond milk
2 heaped tsp crushed garlic
4 tsp almond flour
5 tsp Oryx desert salt
1 tsp ground black pepper
1 Tbsp dried rosemary
6 Tbsp raw honey
zest and juice of 2 lemons
100 g spinach, chopped
4 celery stalks, chopped
4 large carrots, sliced
2 handfuls of chopped fresh
Italian parsley

OVEN-ROASTED CHICKPEAS

2 x 410 g cans chickpeas, drained
1 Tbsp olive oil
½ tsp Oryx desert salt
¼ tsp ground black pepper
1 tsp paprika
pinch of dried parsley

Spray a large saucepan with non-stick cooking spray. Add all the soup ingredients and bring to the boil over low heat, stirring regularly. Cook for about 45 minutes until the vegetables are soft and the soup is lovely and thick.

While the soup is cooking, preheat the oven to 220 °C and spray a baking tray with non-stick cooking spray or line with baking paper.

Rinse the chickpeas and pat dry with paper towel.

Place the chickpeas in a mixing bowl and stir in the oil, salt, black pepper, paprika and parsley.

Spread the chickpeas on the greased baking tray and bake for 15–25 minutes until crispy.

Serve the soup sprinkled with the oven-roasted chickpeas.

NOTE: *Serve with freshly baked rosemary almond bread (see page 33) for a complete meal.*

SERVINGS: 8–10

THAI BUTTERNUT
AND CHICKEN CURRY

1 kg butternut, peeled and chopped
1 Tbsp olive oil
4–5 chicken fillets, chopped
2 medium red onions, diced
1 medium red bell pepper, cut into
strips (keep the seeds)
4 heaped Tbsp mild red curry paste
juice of 1 lime
2 cups unsweetened almond milk
1 Tbsp raw honey
2 tsp Oryx desert salt
½ tsp ground black pepper
½ cup chopped fresh coriander

1. Steam the butternut on the stove or in the microwave until soft.
2. In a large saucepan, heat the olive oil and fry the chicken, onions, bell pepper and reserved seeds until the chicken turns white.
3. Add the red curry paste and mix well, then add the steamed butternut, lime juice, almond milk, honey, salt, black pepper and coriander.
4. Cook for 20–30 minutes until the chicken is tender and the sauce has thickened.

NOTE: *While this recipe is perfect with a mild curry paste, if you'd like extra bite, go for a medium curry paste and add another 1 Tbsp raw honey.*

SERVINGS: 4–6

These are both winning recipes for when you have to cook for a vegetarian and non-vegetarian crowd — one base with two protein options: chicken or chickpeas?!

THAI BUTTERNUT
AND CHICKPEA CURRY

1 kg butternut, peeled and chopped
2 Tbsp olive oil
2 medium red onions, diced
1 medium red bell pepper, cut into
strips (keep the seeds)
4 heaped Tbsp mild red curry paste
juice of 1 lime
2 cups unsweetened almond milk
1 Tbsp raw honey
2 tsp Oryx desert salt
½ tsp ground black pepper
½ cup chopped fresh coriander
2 x 410 g cans chickpeas, drained
and rinsed

Steam the butternut on the stove or in the microwave until soft.
In a large saucepan, heat the olive oil and fry the onions, bell pepper and reserved seeds until the vegetables are soft and almost caramelised.
Add the red curry paste and mix well, then add the steamed butternut, lime juice, almond milk, honey, salt, black pepper and coriander.
Cook for 20 minutes, then add the chickpeas and cook for another 10–15 minutes.

NOTE: *While this recipe is perfect with a mild curry paste, if you'd like extra bite, go for a medium curry paste and add another 1 Tbsp raw honey.*

SERVINGS: 4–6

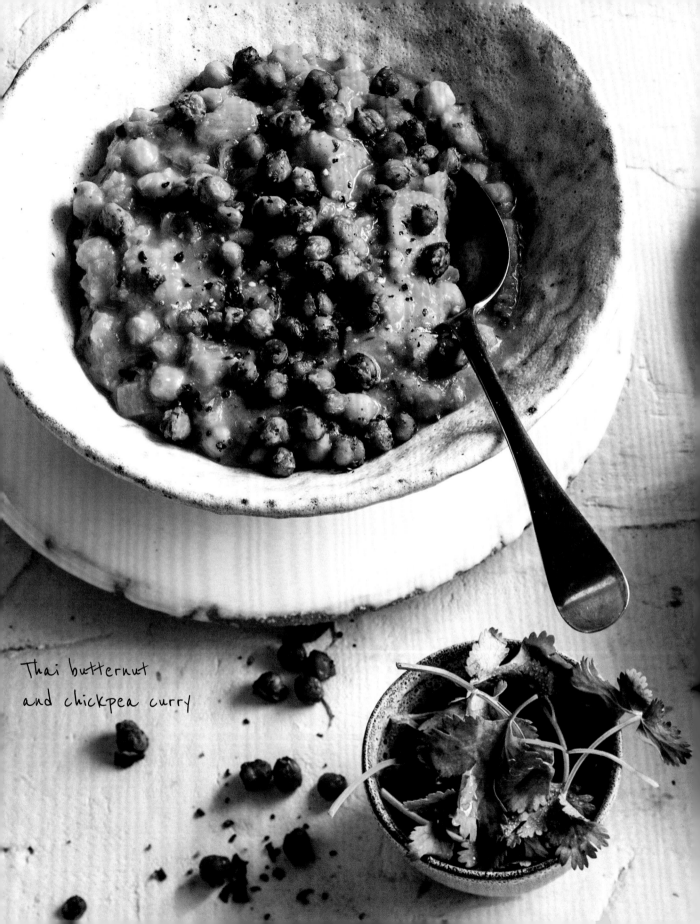

Thai butternut
and chickpea curry

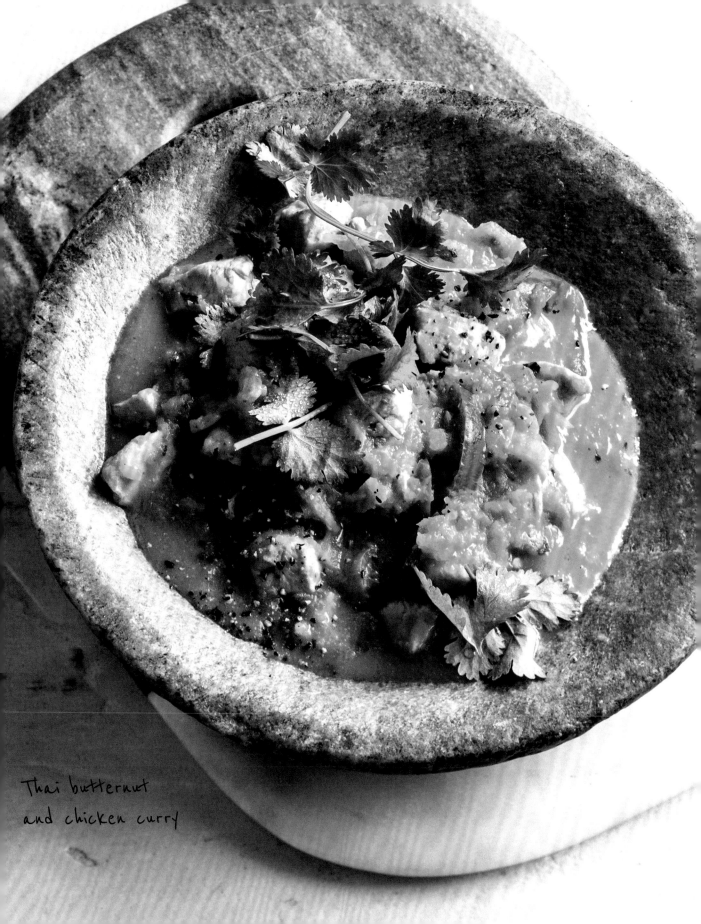

Thai butternut
and chicken curry

FILLET MEDALLIONS WITH CHILLI-CHOCOLATE SAUCE

400 g fillet medallions
1 Tbsp olive oil
Oryx desert salt and ground black pepper
chopped fresh thyme for garnishing

CHILLI-CHOCOLATE SAUCE

1 Tbsp olive oil
150 ml unsweetened almond milk
120 g almond butter
3 Tbsp raw honey
2 heaped Tbsp raw cacao powder
¼ tsp Oryx desert salt
1 tsp caramel essence
1 fresh red chilli, deseeded and chopped
1 tsp balsamic vinegar

1. First make the sauce. Spray a small saucepan with non-stick cooking spray. Add all the ingredients and heat up over low heat. Stir until the sauce thickens.
2. Rub the fillet medallions with the olive oil and season with salt and black pepper. Cook to preference.
3. Pour the sauce over the meat, garnish with fresh thyme and serve immediately with thinly sliced oven-grilled sweet potato crisps seasoned with olive oil, salt and black pepper.

NOTE: *To make sweet potato crisps, cut whole sweet potatoes into thin chips. Preheat the oven to 200 °C and spray a baking tray with non-stick cooking spray or line with baking paper. Place the sweet potato chips on the tray and drizzle with olive oil. Season with salt and black pepper and bake until desired crispiness.*

SERVINGS: 2

The perfect dinner for two xxx

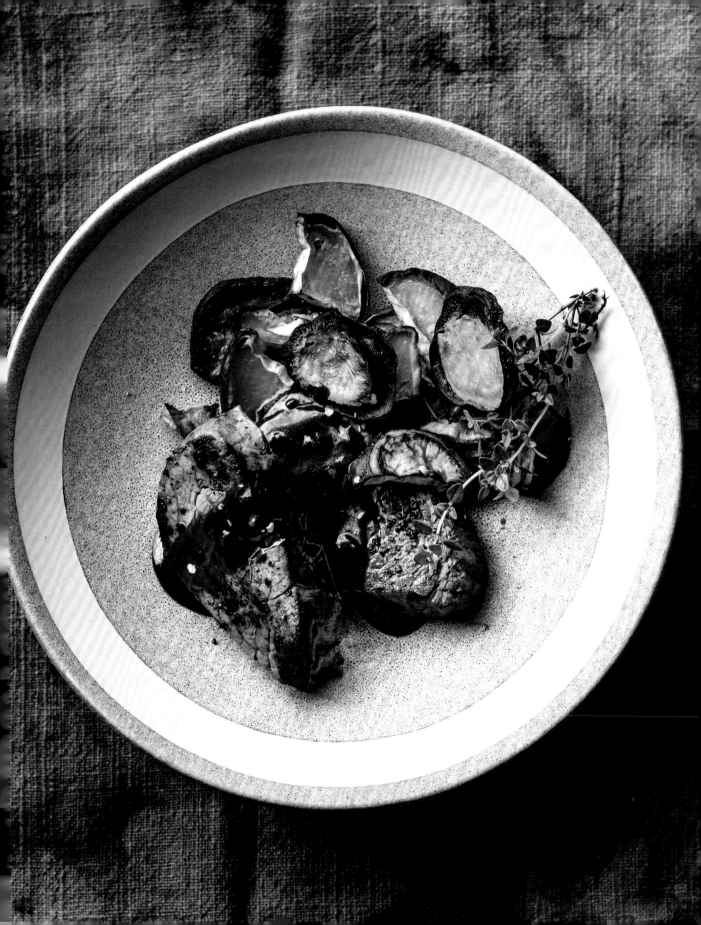

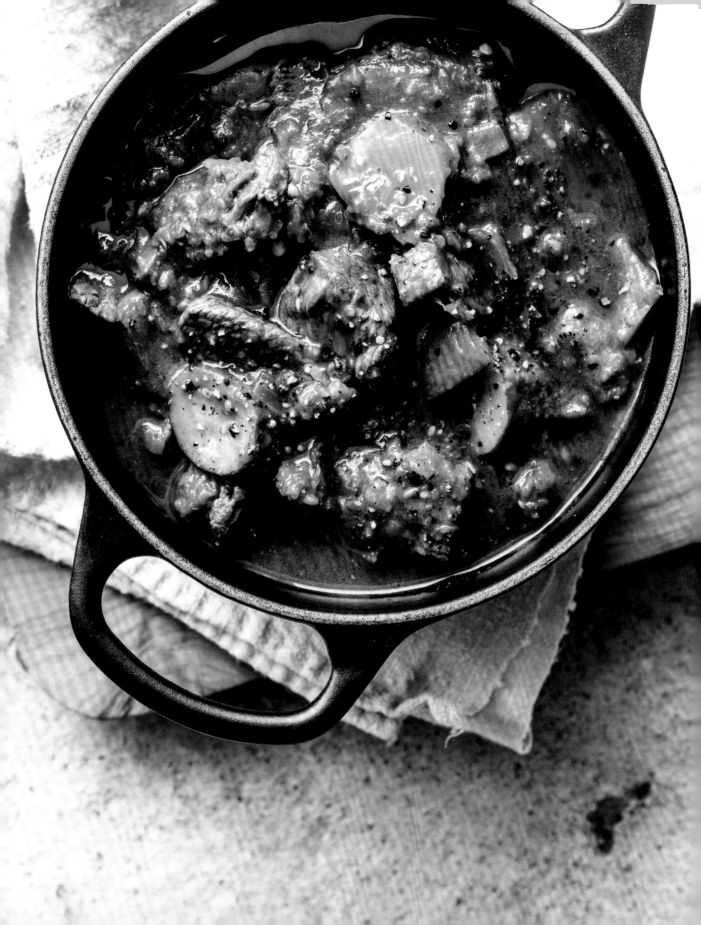

Inspired by Dad's goulash recipe — the rest is history

BEEF GOULASH

1 Tbsp olive oil
2 red onions, diced
1 small green bell pepper, cut into strips (keep the seeds)
1.6 kg lean beef cubes
1 Tbsp Oryx desert wine salt
2½ heaped Tbsp paprika
5 Tbsp balsamic vinegar
¼ cup raw honey
1 Tbsp dried parsley
750 g rosa tomatoes, halved
1 kg pkt mixed potjie vegetables
650 ml boiling water
¼ cup chopped fresh parsley

Heat the olive oil in a large saucepan and fry the onions, bell pepper, reserved seeds and beef cubes until the meat is browned.

Season with the salt, paprika, balsamic vinegar, honey and dried parsley. Stir well.

Spray a separate saucepan with non-stick cooking spray and cook the rosa tomatoes for about 10 minutes until they are a stew-like consistency, then add to the meat.

Cut a corner off the packet of potjie vegetables and microwave on high for 15 minutes.

Add the steamed potjie vegetables and boiling water to the meat and cook for 20–25 minutes until most of the water has evaporated.

Garnish with the fresh parsley before serving with parsley-flavoured basmati rice or oven-roasted corn on the cob.

SERVINGS: 6

VEGETARIAN CHICKPEA GOULASH

1 Tbsp olive oil
1 medium red onion, diced
100 g green bell pepper, cut into
strips (keep the seeds)
1 Tbsp Oryx desert wine salt
2 heaped Tbsp paprika
¼ cup balsamic vinegar
3 Tbsp raw honey
2 tsp dried parsley
500 g rosa tomatoes, halved
300 g carrots, chopped
300 g green beans, chopped
200 g sweet potato, cut into chunks
4 cups boiling water
4 x 410 g cans chickpeas, drained
and rinsed
¼ cup chopped fresh parsley

1. Heat the olive oil in a medium saucepan and fry the onion, bell pepper and reserved seeds until soft.
2. Add the salt, paprika, balsamic vinegar, honey and dried parsley. Stir well.
3. Add the rosa tomatoes, carrots, green beans, sweet potato and boiling water and cook for 15–20 minutes or until most of the water has evaporated.
4. Add the chickpeas, stir well and allow to cook for 5–10 minutes. You can add another cup of water at this point if you prefer it saucier.
5. Garnish with the fresh parsley before serving with your choice of basmati or brown rice, baked potato or sweet potato, couscous or quinoa.

SERVINGS: 6

For vegetarians and meat-free Mondays!
xxx

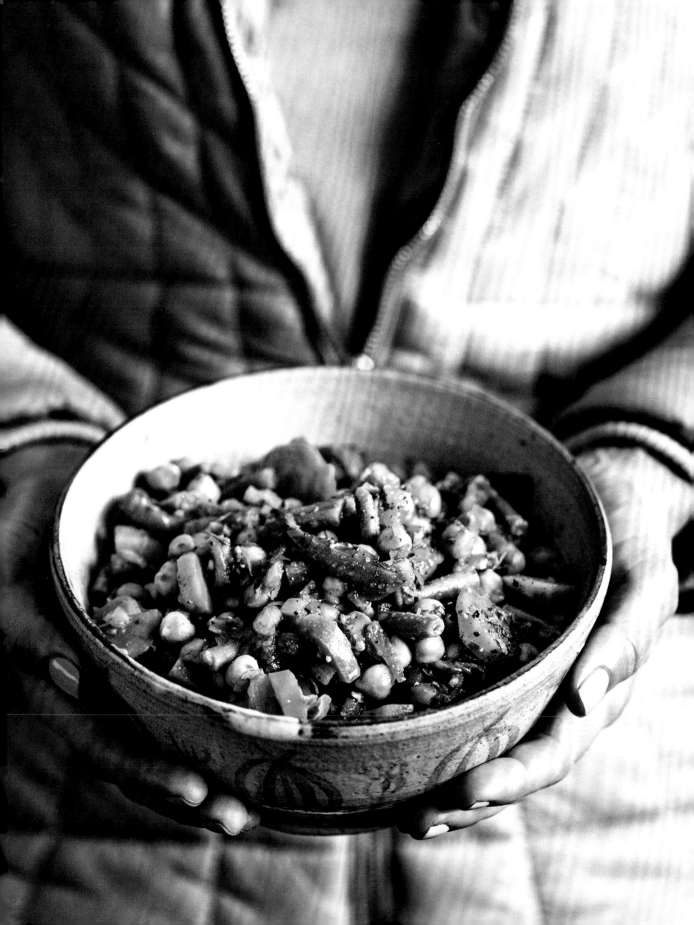

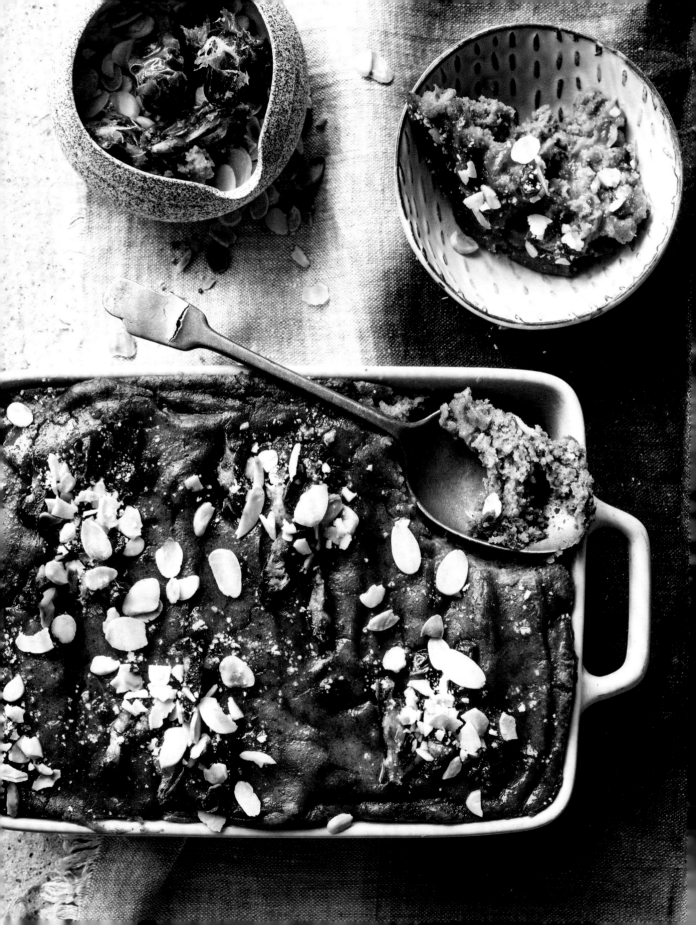

CARAMEL DATE PUDDING

2 x 410 g cans chickpeas, drained
and rinsed
6 Tbsp raw honey
100 g almond butter
1 tsp vanilla essence
2 tsp caramel essence
1 tsp bicarbonate of soda
1 tsp ground cinnamon (optional)
90 g almond flour
100 g pitted dates, chopped
1 tsp Oryx desert salt
2 jumbo eggs

SAUCE

200 g almond butter
6 Tbsp raw honey
2 tsp caramel essence
1½ cups unsweetened almond milk
1 tsp Oryx desert salt
50 g pitted dates, chopped

TOPPING

handful of flaked almonds
2 pitted dates, chopped
½ tsp almond flour

Preheat the oven to 180 °C on thermo-fan and spray a 20 x 30 cm ovenproof dish with non-stick cooking spray.

Place the chickpeas in the bowl of a food processor and blend until smooth. Add the rest of the ingredients, except the eggs, and process on high for 3–5 minutes, scraping down the sides, until the mixture is smooth and well blended. (If you don't have a food processor, you can pulp the chickpeas with a blender, add the rest of the ingredients and beat with an electric beater for 2 minutes on high speed.)

Beat the eggs in a separate bowl until light and fluffy, then add to the chickpea mixture and beat for another 30 seconds to mix well.

Scoop the mixture into the prepared dish and bake for 20 minutes.

To make the sauce, spray a small saucepan with non-stick cooking spray. Add all the ingredients and cook over medium heat until the almond butter starts to melt. The sauce will get a glazed look and have a slightly toasted nutty/caramel flavour.

After 20 minutes, remove the pudding from the oven and pour over the sauce. Top with the flaked almonds and chopped dates and dust with the almond flour. Bake for another 10 minutes.

Serve warm.

SERVINGS: 6–8

For a festive twist, add 100 g cranberries to the mix – be on the lookout for ones sweetened with pineapple juice

For the love of raw cacao!

STICKY CHOCOLATE PUDDING

2 x 410 g cans chickpeas, drained
and rinsed
½ cup raw honey
100 g almond butter
1 tsp vanilla essence
2 tsp caramel essence
1 tsp bicarbonate of soda
50 g almond flour
1 tsp Oryx desert salt
1 heaped Tbsp raw cacao powder,
plus extra for dusting
2 eggs
fresh mint for garnishing (optional)

SAUCE

200 g almond butter
1½ cups unsweetened almond milk
5 Tbsp raw honey
1 heaped Tbsp raw cacao powder
pinch of Oryx desert salt
1 tsp caramel essence
1 fresh red chilli, deseeded and
chopped (optional for a
chilli-chocolate sauce)
1 tsp balsamic vinegar (optional for a
chilli-chocolate sauce)

1. Preheat the oven to 180 °C on thermo-fan and spray a 20 x 30 cm ovenproof dish with non-stick cooking spray.
2. Place the chickpeas in the bowl of a food processor and blend until smooth. Add the rest of the ingredients, except the eggs and mint, and process on high for 3–5 minutes, scraping down the sides, until the mixture is smooth and well blended. (If you don't have a food processor, you can pulp the chickpeas with a blender, add the rest of the ingredients and beat with an electric beater for 2 minutes on high speed.)
3. Beat the eggs in a separate bowl until light and fluffy, then add to the chickpea mixture and beat for another 30 seconds to mix well.
4. Pour the mixture into the prepared dish and bake for 10 minutes.
5. To make the sauce, spray a small saucepan with non-stick cooking spray. Add all the ingredients and cook over medium heat until the almond butter starts to melt. The sauce will get a glazed look and have a slightly toasted nutty flavour.
6. After 10 minutes, remove the pudding from the oven, pour over the sauce and then bake for another 10–15 minutes. When done, the edges of the pudding will be crispy and firm to the touch, while the centre will remain moist and soft.
7. Serve warm, dusted with cacao powder and garnished with fresh mint if desired.

SERVINGS: 6—8

Transform this decadent dessert into a chilli-chocolate sensation by adding red chilli and balsamic vinegar to the sauce

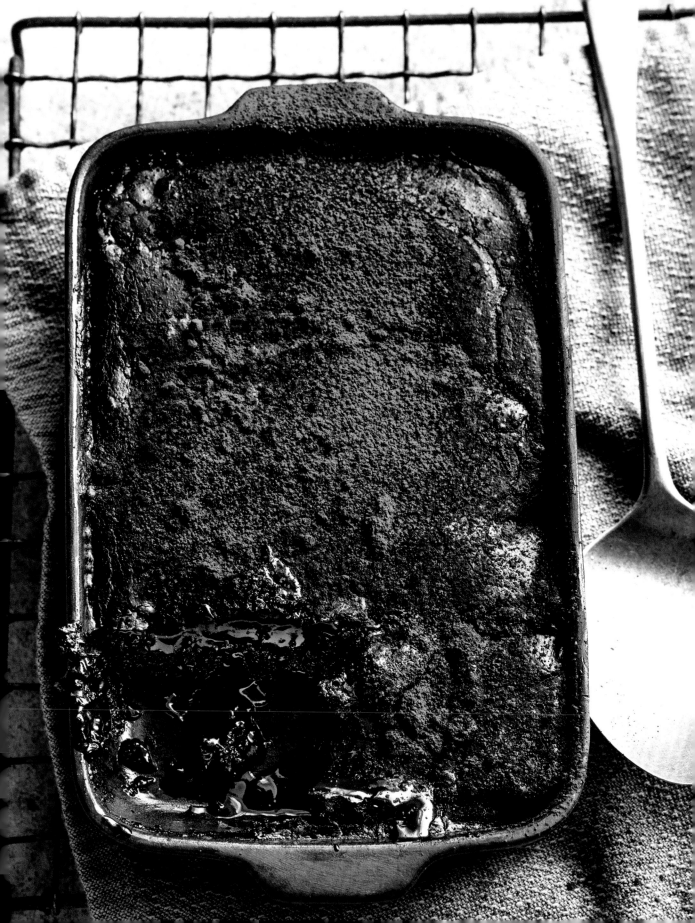

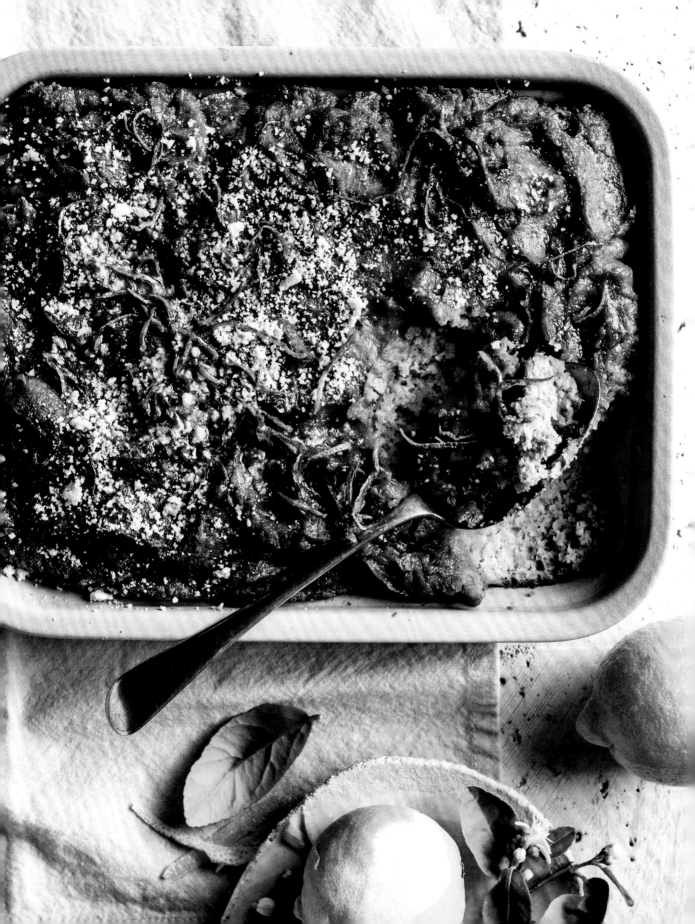

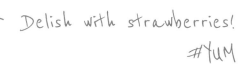

Delish with strawberries!
#YUM

LEMON PUDDING

2 x 410 g cans chickpeas, drained and rinsed
6 Tbsp raw honey
100 g almond butter
1 tsp vanilla essence
2 tsp caramel essence
1 tsp bicarbonate of soda
100 g almond flour
1 tsp Oryx desert salt
1 heaped Tbsp lemon zest
juice of 1 lemon
2 eggs

SAUCE
200 g almond butter
6 Tbsp raw honey
2 tsp caramel essence
1½ cups unsweetened almond milk
1 tsp Oryx desert salt
juice of 1 lemon

TOPPING
chopped peel of 1 lemon fried in olive oil, honey and salt until golden brown
raw honey for drizzling
almond flour for dusting

Preheat the oven to 180 °C on thermo-fan and spray a 20 x 30 cm ovenproof dish with non-stick cooking spray.

Place the chickpeas in the bowl of a food processor and blend until smooth. Add the rest of the ingredients, except the eggs, and process on high for 3–5 minutes, scraping down the sides, until the mixture is smooth and well blended. (If you don't have a food processor, you can pulp the chickpeas with a blender, add the rest of the ingredients and beat with an electric beater for 2 minutes on high speed.)

Beat the eggs in a separate bowl until light and fluffy, then add to the chickpea mixture and beat for another 30 seconds to mix well.

Scoop the mixture into the prepared dish and bake for 20 minutes.

To make the sauce, spray a small saucepan with non-stick cooking spray. Add all the ingredients, except the lemon juice, and cook over medium heat until the almond butter starts to melt. Bring to the boil and allow to thicken, stirring continuously. The sauce will get a glazed look and have a slightly toasted nutty flavour. Stir in the lemon juice.

After 20 minutes, remove the pudding from the oven and scoop over the sauce. Top with the fried lemon peel and a drizzle of honey. Bake for another 15 minutes.

Serve warm, dusted with almond flour.

NOTE: *This delish dessert is light and fluffy, and ideal after a lunch or dinner with a lot of red meat because of the alkalising elements it contains.*

SERVINGS: 6–8

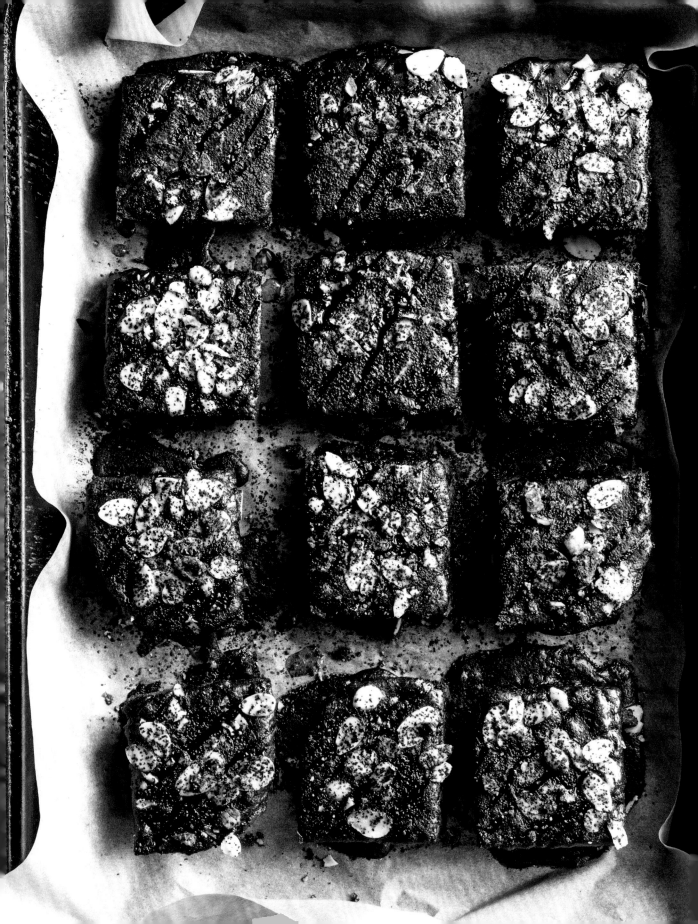

YOU ONLY LIVE ONCE ... so eat that cake!

Cake, biscuits, smoothies, desserts ... they aren't usually best friends with your waistline and thighs, but stop the bus, drop off that perception and change your mindset immediately, because these recipes are not only life changers, but also perception changers! So have your cake and eat it ... guilt free!

SWEET POTATO CHOCOLATE BROWNIES

1 kg sweet potato, peeled and chopped
100 g almond flour
2 heaped Tbsp raw cacao powder
5 Tbsp raw honey
2 tsp vanilla essence
2 tsp caramel essence
1 tsp Oryx desert salt
2 tsp bicarbonate of soda
4 whole eggs
4 egg whites

ICING

300 g almond or macadamia butter
5 Tbsp raw honey
1 heaped Tbsp raw cacao powder
pinch of Oryx desert salt
1 tsp caramel essence

TOPPING

flaked almonds (or pecans, hazelnuts or macadamias, or chopped dates and a grind of Oryx desert salt)
raw honey
raw cacao powder
fresh mint leaves (optional)

Preheat the oven to 180 °C and spray a 20 x 30 cm ovenproof dish with non-stick cooking spray or line it with baking paper.

Steam the sweet potato until soft, drain and place in a mixing bowl. Mash until smooth.

Add the almond flour, cacao powder, honey, vanilla essence, caramel essence, salt and bicarbonate of soda. Beat to an even texture.

In a separate mixing bowl, beat the whole eggs and egg whites until fluffy – this is important, as it influences the texture of the brownie. Add the beaten eggs to the sweet potato mixture and continue beating to a mousse-like texture.

Pour the batter into the prepared dish and bake for 30 minutes.

To make the icing, mix all the ingredients until smooth.

After 30 minutes, remove the brownie from the oven and spread with the icing. Sprinkle over flaked almonds, drizzle with honey and dust with cacao powder.

Return to the oven and bake for another 20 minutes. Allow to cool in the dish before cutting into squares. Garnish with fresh mint before serving if desired. As these are very moist, it's best to store them in the fridge.

SERVINGS: 12 BROWNIES

Most irresistible after 2 days in the fridge or straight from the oven

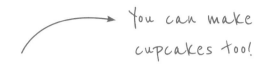
You can make cupcakes too!

ALMOND BUTTER CAKE

2 x 410 g cans chickpeas, drained
and rinsed
6 Tbsp raw honey
100 g almond butter
1 tsp vanilla essence
2 tsp caramel essence
1 tsp bicarbonate of soda
90 g almond flour
1 tsp Oryx desert salt
2 jumbo eggs

ICING

300 g almond butter
6 Tbsp raw honey
2 tsp caramel essence
½ cup unsweetened almond milk
1 tsp Oryx desert salt

TOPPING

whole blanched almonds
fresh berries
sliced fresh figs
almond flour for dusting

1. Preheat the oven to 180 °C on thermo-fan. Line a 23 cm springform cake pan with baking paper and then spray with non-stick cooking spray. Alternatively, line a cupcake pan with paper cupcake liners sprayed with non-stick cooking spray.
2. Place the chickpeas in the bowl of a food processor and blend until smooth. Add the rest of the ingredients, except the eggs, and process on high for 3–5 minutes, scraping down the sides, until the batter is smooth and well blended. (If you don't have a food processor, you can pulp the chickpeas with a blender, add the rest of the ingredients and beat with an electric beater for 2 minutes on high speed.)
3. Beat the eggs in a separate bowl until light and fluffy, then add to the batter and beat for another 30 seconds to mix well.
4. Pour the batter into the prepared cake or cupcake pan and bake for 25–30 minutes. The edges will be crispy and firm to the touch, while the centre will remain moist and soft. Remove from the oven and allow to cool slightly in the pan before turning out onto a wire rack.
5. To make the icing, spray a small saucepan with non-stick cooking spray. Add all the ingredients and cook over medium heat until the almond butter starts to melt. The icing will get a glazed look and have a slightly toasted nutty flavour.
6. Apply the warm icing to the cooled cake or cupcakes – you want the icing to cool on the cake to give it that glazed, smooth look. Garnish with blanched almonds, fresh berries and fresh figs as desired and dust with almond flour.

NOTE: *This recipe makes a single-layer cake. To make a double-layer cake, simply double up the cake ingredients.*

SERVINGS: 1 CAKE OR 12 CUPCAKES

Replace the berries with pineapple for a delish alternative #winningatlife

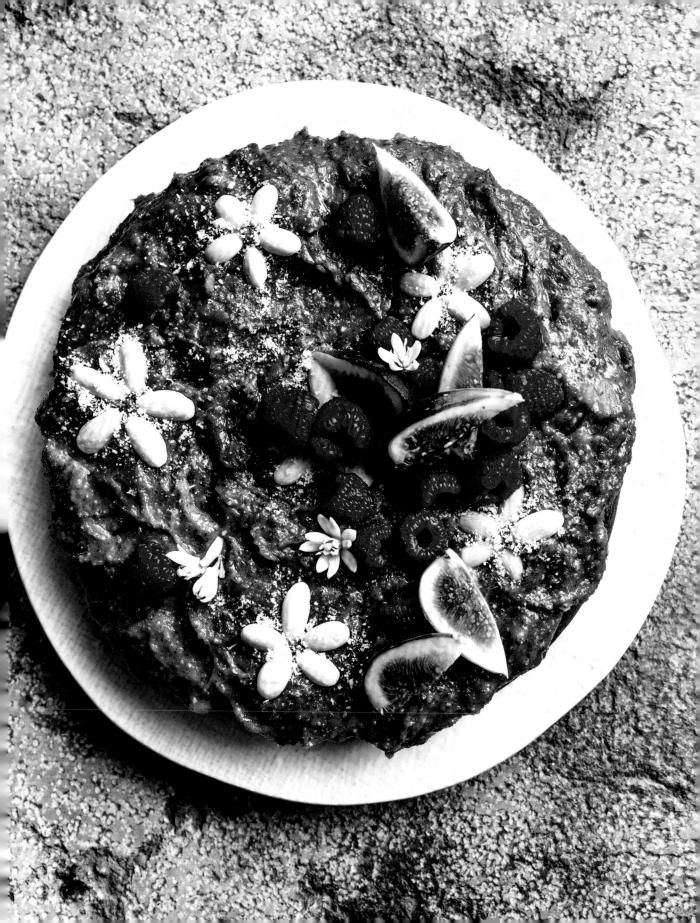

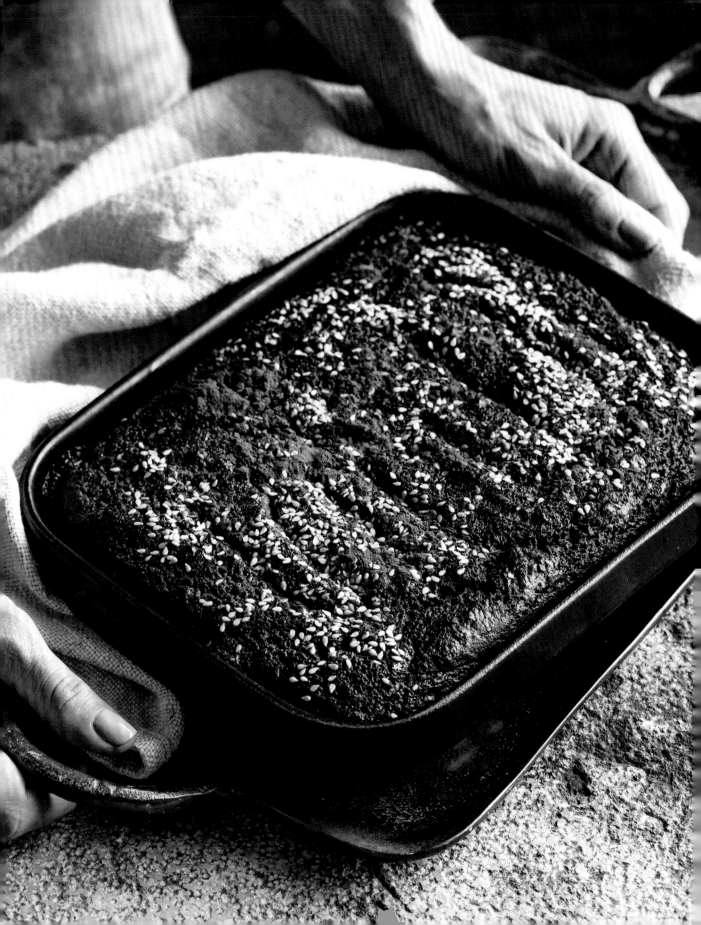

GINGER BISCUIT BAKE

500 g steamed and mashed sweet
potato or butternut
300 g almond flour
50 g tahini
2 tsp bicarbonate of soda
2 tsp ground cinnamon, plus extra
for dusting
4 tsp ground ginger
1 tsp ground cloves
1 tsp Oryx desert salt
1 tsp vanilla essence
2 Tbsp blackstrap molasses
3 Tbsp raw honey, plus extra
for drizzling
3 large eggs
sesame seeds for garnishing

Preheat the oven to 200 °C and spray a 20 x 30 cm ovenproof dish with non-stick cooking spray.

Combine all the ingredients, except the eggs and sesame seeds, and mix well.

Beat the eggs in a separate bowl until fluffy, then add to the mixture and beat for about 1 minute.

Pour into the prepared dish, garnish with sesame seeds, a drizzle of honey and a dusting of cinnamon and bake for 40 minutes.

Serve warm or cold.

NOTE: *This is the perfect guilt-free dessert loaded with iron and magnesium.*

SERVINGS: 6−8

One of my favourite biscuits in the form of a bake! :-D

This recipe is perfect for making mini ginger loaves as well (just reduce baking time to 30 minutes)

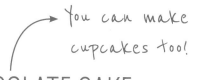
You can make cupcakes too!

GUILT-FREE CHOCOLATE CAKE

2 x 410 g cans chickpeas, drained and rinsed
½ cup raw honey
100 g almond butter
1 tsp vanilla essence
2 tsp caramel essence
1 tsp bicarbonate of soda
50 g almond flour
I tsp Oryx desert salt
1 heaped Tbsp raw cacao powder
2 eggs

ICING

250 g almond butter
100 ml unsweetened almond milk
5 Tbsp raw honey
1 heaped Tbsp raw cacao powder
pinch of Oryx desert salt
1 tsp caramel essence
4–6 drops peppermint essence (optional for a mint-chocolate cake)

TOPPING

chopped almonds (or pecans or hazelnuts, or chopped dates and a grind of Oryx desert salt)
fresh berries, edible glitter and fresh mint (optional)

1. Preheat the oven to 180 °C on thermo-fan. Line a 23 cm springform cake pan with baking paper and then spray with non-stick cooking spray. Alternatively, line a cupcake pan with paper cupcake liners sprayed with non-stick cooking spray.
2. Place the chickpeas in the bowl of a food processor and blend until smooth. Add all the other ingredients, except the eggs, and process on high for 3–5 minutes, scraping down the sides, until the batter is smooth and well blended. (If you don't have a food processor, you can pulp the chickpeas with a blender, add the rest of the ingredients and beat with an electric beater for 2 minutes on high speed.)
3. Beat the eggs in a separate bowl until light and fluffy, then add to the batter and beat for another 30 seconds to mix well.
4. Pour the batter into the prepared cake or cupcake pan and bake for 20–25 minutes. The edges will be crispy and firm to the touch, while the centre will remain moist and soft. Remove from the oven and allow to cool slightly in the pan before turning out onto a wire rack.
5. To make the icing, spray a small saucepan with non-stick cooking spray. Add all the ingredients and cook over medium heat until the almond butter starts to melt. The icing will get a glazed look and have a slightly toasted nutty flavour.
6. Apply the warm icing to the cooled cake or cupcakes – you want the icing to cool on the cake to give it that glazed, smooth look. Top with chopped almonds, fresh berries, edible glitter and fresh mint as desired.

NOTE: *This recipe makes a single-layer cake. To make a double-layer cake, simply double up the cake ingredients.*

SERVINGS: 1 CAKE OR 12 CUPCAKES

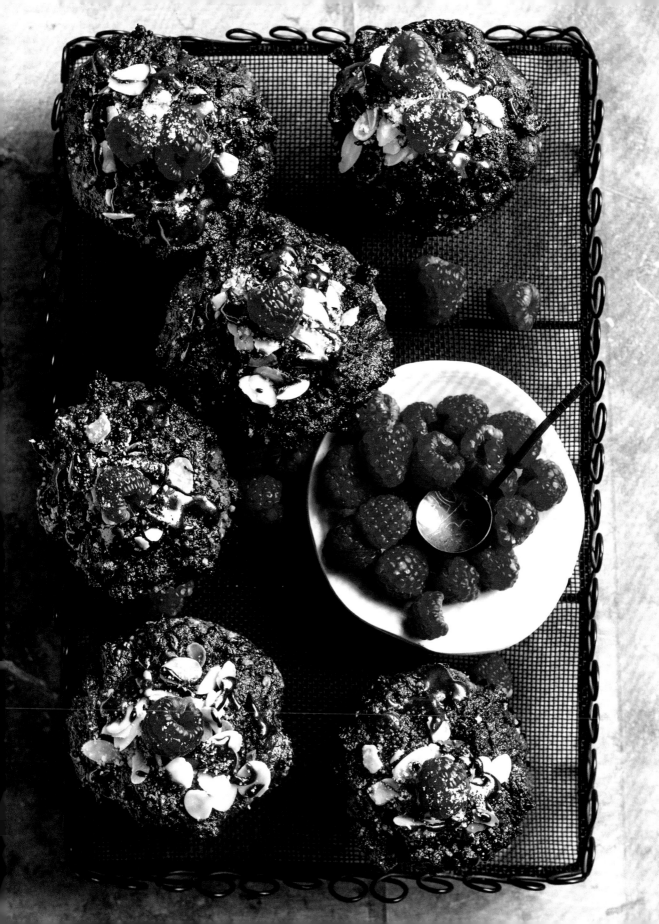

ALMOND APPLE CRUMBLE

FILLING

2 x 385 g cans unsweetened
pie apples
100 g raisins
1 tsp caramel essence
¼ tsp Oryx desert salt
½ tsp ground nutmeg
1 tsp ground cinnamon

CRUMBLE

120 g almond flour, plus 1 Tbsp extra
for dusting
50 g flaked almonds
50 g pitted dates, chopped
1 tsp ground cinnamon
½ tsp Oryx desert salt
100 g almond butter, melted
2 Tbsp raw honey
1 tsp vanilla essence

TOPPING

thinly sliced fresh apple
raw honey for drizzling
almond flour for dusting

1. Preheat the oven to 180 °C. Spray a 23 cm pie dish with non-stick cooking spray and dust with 1 Tbsp almond flour.
2. In a large mixing bowl, combine all the filling ingredients. Transfer to the prepared dish, spread out evenly and press down gently.
3. Place all the crumble ingredients in another mixing bowl and, using your fingertips, rub until the mixture has a large crumb-like texture.
4. Sprinkle the crumble over the apple filling and bake for 20–25 minutes. Remove from the oven, top with fresh apple slices, drizzle over some honey and dust with almond flour. Bake for another 5–10 minutes.
5. Serve warm or cool.

SERVING: 6—8

For that special occasion!

ALMOND BLUEBERRY CRUMBLE

FILLING
400 g fresh or defrosted
frozen blueberries
¼ tsp Oryx desert salt
1 tsp caramel essence

CRUMBLE
120 g almond flour, plus 1 Tbsp extra
for dusting
50 g flaked almonds
50 g pitted dates, chopped
1 tsp ground cinnamon
½ tsp Oryx desert salt
100 g almond butter, melted
2 Tbsp raw honey, plus extra
for drizzling
1 tsp vanilla essence

Preheat the oven to 180 °C. Spray a 23 cm pie dish with non-stick cooking spray and dust with 1 Tbsp almond flour.

In a large mixing bowl, combine all the filling ingredients. Transfer to the prepared dish, spread out evenly and press down gently.

Place all the crumble ingredients in another mixing bowl and, using your fingertips, rub until the mixture has a large crumb-like texture.

Sprinkle the crumble over the blueberry filling and bake for 20–25 minutes. Remove from the oven, drizzle over some honey and bake for another 5–10 minutes.

Serve warm or cool.

SERVING: 6–8

Add some freshly cut dessert peach slices to the blueberries before covering with crumble for a peach & blueberry alternative (use 1 large or 2 small peaches)

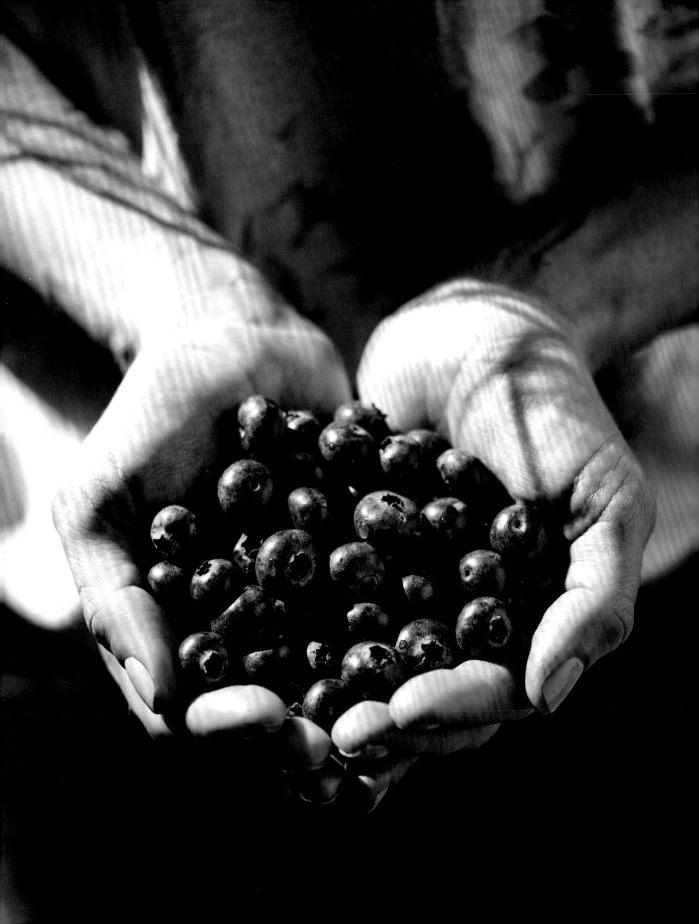

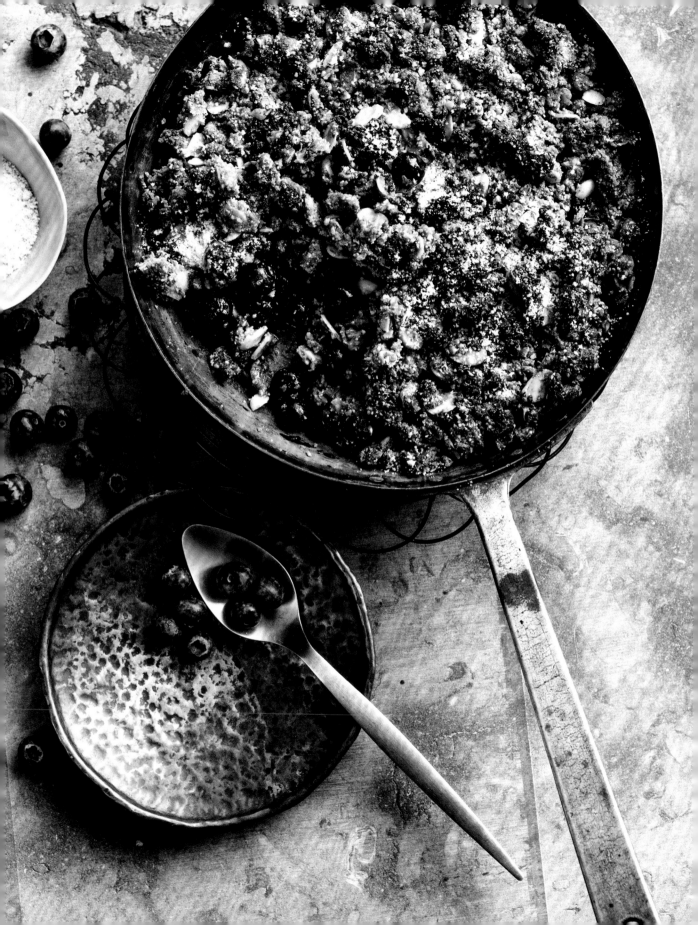

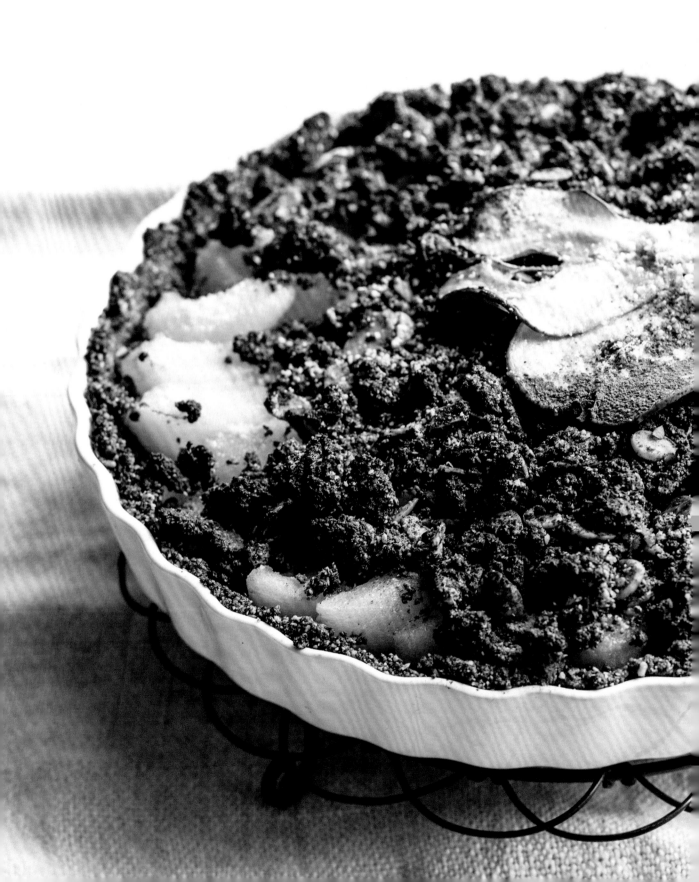

Even better the next day

CHOCOLATE PEAR CRUMBLE

CRUST

250 g almond flour
2 Tbsp raw honey
1 Tbsp water
1 tsp Oryx desert salt
1 heaped tsp raw cacao powder
1 tsp caramel essence

FILLING

3 x 410 g cans pear halves in fruit
juice (Lite), drained and rinsed
½ tsp Oryx desert salt
1 Tbsp caramel essence
thinly sliced fresh pear for garnishing

CRUMBLE

120 g almond flour
50 g flaked almonds
50 g pitted dates, chopped
1 tsp ground cinnamon, plus extra
for dusting
1 tsp Oryx desert salt
100 g almond butter, melted
2 Tbsp raw honey, plus extra
for drizzling
1 tsp caramel essence
1 tsp vanilla essence
1 heaped Tbsp raw cacao powder

Preheat the oven to 180 °C and spray a 23 cm pie dish with non-stick cooking spray.

In a large mixing bowl, mix all the crust ingredients to a sticky crumb. Tip into the prepared dish, spread evenly and press down firmly using your hands.

Cut the pear halves into smaller pieces (depending on the size of your serving dish) and place in a clean mixing bowl with the salt and caramel essence. Mix well to coat, then spoon onto the crust and spread evenly.

Place all the crumble ingredients in another mixing bowl and rub until the mixture has a sticky crumb-like texture.

Sprinkle the crumble over the pear filling, garnish with thinly sliced fresh pear, drizzle with honey and dust with cinnamon. Bake for 25–30 minutes. Serve warm or cool.

SERVINGS: 6–8

To transform this scrumptious bake into a mint-chocolate pear sensation, add 4–6 drops peppermint essence to the crumble and thank me later!
#ThanksCarl

LEMON CHIA SEED MUFFINS

2 x 410 g cans chickpeas, drained
and rinsed
6 Tbsp raw honey, plus extra
for topping
100 g almond butter
1 tsp vanilla essence
2 tsp caramel essence
1 tsp bicarbonate of soda
100 g almond flour, plus extra
for topping
1 tsp Oryx desert salt
1 heaped Tbsp lemon zest, plus extra
for topping
juice of 1 lemon
2 heaped Tbsp chia seeds
2 eggs

1. Preheat the oven to 180 °C on thermo-fan and line a muffin pan with paper muffin liners.
2. Place the chickpeas in the bowl of a food processor and blend until smooth. Add all the other ingredients, except the eggs, and process on high for 3–5 minutes, scraping down the sides, until the mixture is smooth and well blended. (If you don't have a food processor, you can pulp the chickpeas with a blender, add the rest of the ingredients and beat with an electric beater for 2 minutes on high speed.)
3. Beat the eggs in a separate bowl until light and fluffy, then add to the mixture and beat for another 30 seconds to mix well.
4. Scoop the mixture into the prepared muffin cups and top each with a sprinkle of extra lemon zest, almond flour and a drizzle of honey for a beautiful caramelised look.
5. Bake for 25–30 minutes. The edges will be crispy and firm to the touch while the centres will remain moist and soft.

SERVINGS: 12 MUFFINS

Always a crowd-pleaser!

MOCHA HAZELNUT MUFFINS

2 x 410 g cans chickpeas, drained
and rinsed
½ cup raw honey
100 g almond butter
1 tsp vanilla essence
2 tsp caramel essence
1 tsp bicarbonate of soda
50 g almond flour
1 tsp Oryx desert salt
1 heaped Tbsp raw cacao powder
1 shot espresso or 1 heaped tsp
ground or instant coffee
2 eggs
100 g hazelnuts

TOPPING

24-36 hazelnuts
24-36 coffee beans (optional)
almond flour for dusting
raw honey for drizzling

Preheat the oven to 180 °C on thermo-fan and line a muffin pan with paper muffin liners.

Place the chickpeas in the bowl of a food processor and blend until smooth. Add all the other ingredients, except the eggs and hazelnuts, and process on high for 3–5 minutes, scraping down the sides, until the mixture is smooth and well blended. (If you don't have a food processor, you can pulp the chickpeas with a blender, add the rest of the ingredients and beat with an electric beater for 2 minutes on high speed.)

Beat the eggs in a separate bowl until light and fluffy, then add to the mixture and beat for another 30 seconds to mix well. Fold in the hazelnuts.

Scoop the mixture into the prepared muffin cups and top each with 2–3 extra hazelnuts and/or coffee beans, a dusting of almond flour and a drizzle of honey for a beautiful caramelised look.

Bake for 20–25 minutes. The edges will be crispy and firm to the touch while the centres will remain moist and soft.

SERVINGS: 12 MUFFINS

Add a handful of cranberries to the dry
ingredients for a decadent twist!

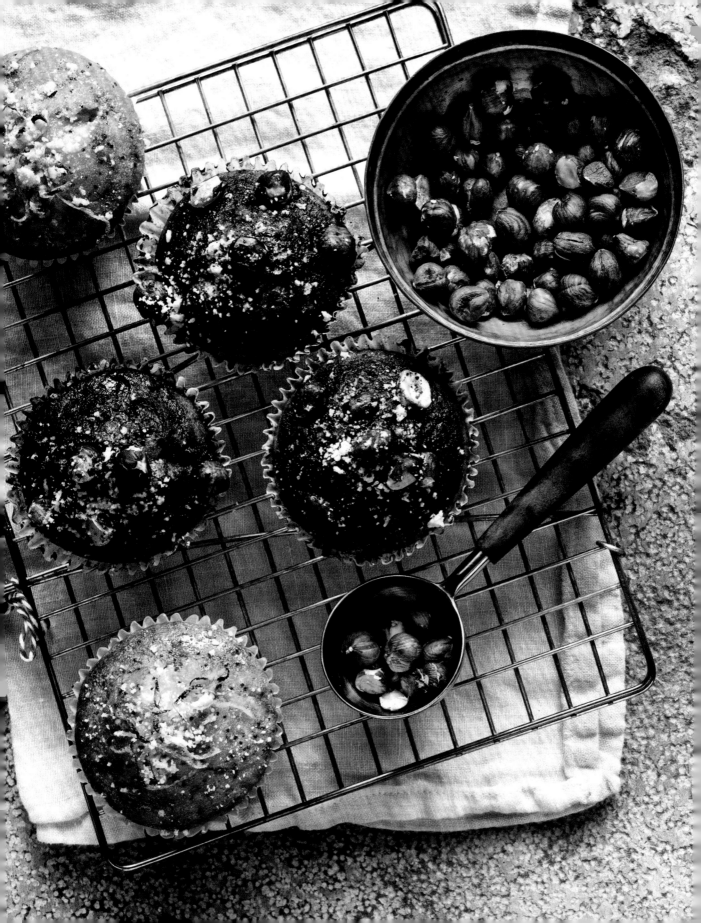

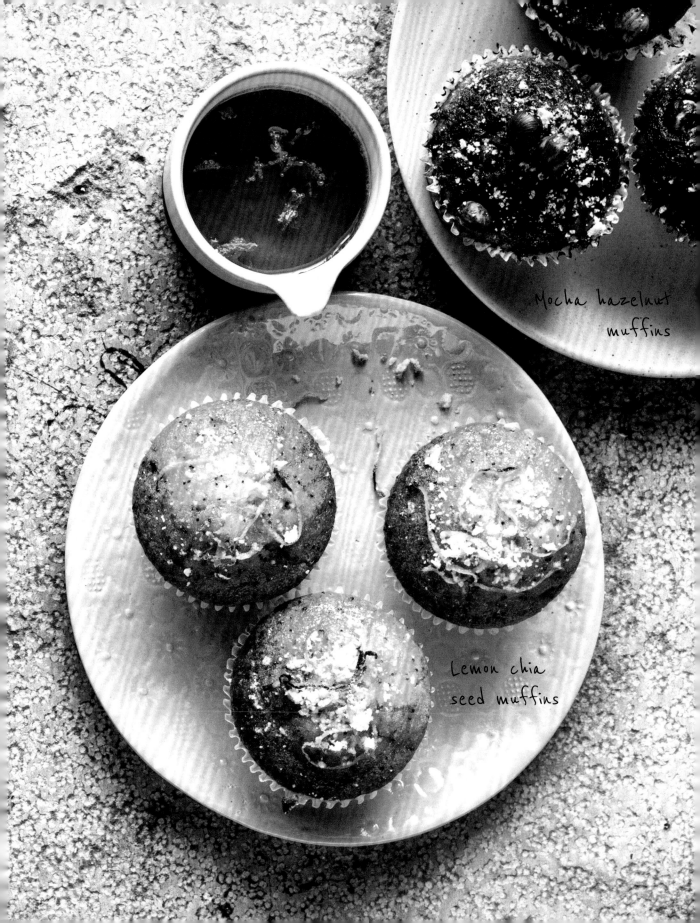

Mocha hazelnut
muffins

Lemon chia
seed muffins

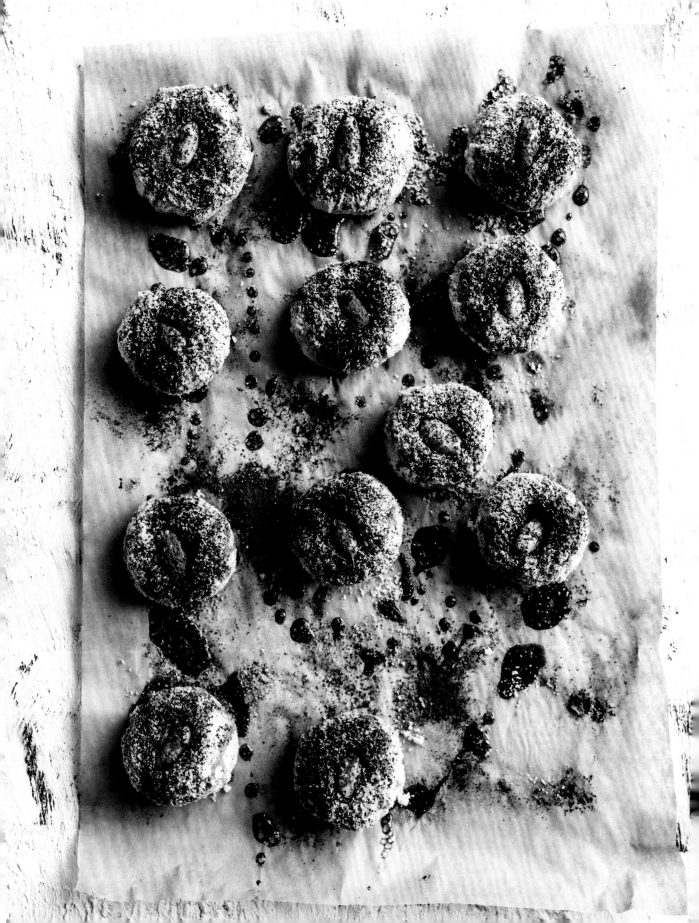

Tastes like 'home' on a cold winter's day!

BAKED RAISIN AND DATE BROWNIE BISCUITS

300 g pitted dates, chopped
300 g raisins
150 g almond flour, plus ½ cup extra for rolling
1 Tbsp caramel essence
¼ cup raw cacao powder
1 tsp ground cinnamon, plus extra for dusting
pinch of Oryx desert salt
50 g whole almonds, roasted
2 tsp raw honey

Preheat the oven to 190 °C. Line a baking tray with foil and spray with non-stick cooking spray.

Soak the dates and raisins in enough hot water to cover for 10–15 minutes. Drain and mash in a mixing bowl.

Add the almond flour, caramel essence, cacao powder, cinnamon and salt and mix well to form a soft dough.

Using your hands, roll a heaped tablespoon of the dough into a ball, flatten it out and place a roasted almond in the middle. Roll it back into a ball and then roll it in the extra almond flour. To prevent the dough sticking to your hands, spray your hands with non-stick cooking spray. Once they start to get sticky, wash your hands and spray again.

Place the dough ball on the prepared baking tray, flatten slightly and place another roasted almond on top. Repeat with the remainder of the dough.

Drizzle the biscuits with the honey, dust with cinnamon and bake for 10–15 minutes. They are meant to be soft and chewy.

Remove from the oven and allow to cool before storing in an airtight container in the fridge.

SERVING: 20 BISCUITS

Swap the almonds for pecan nuts

CHOCOLATE ESPRESSO BISCUITS

300 g almond flour, plus extra
for dusting
50 g diced almonds
1 heaped Tbsp raw cacao powder,
plus extra for dusting
1 tsp fine Oryx desert salt
1 tsp bicarbonate of soda
200 g almond butter
6 Tbsp raw honey, plus extra
for drizzling
2 tsp vanilla essence
1 shot strong espresso or 1 heaped
tsp ground or instant coffee
coffee beans and hazelnuts
or macadamia nuts for
garnishing (optional)

1. Preheat the oven to 200 °C. Spray a baking tray with non-stick cooking spray and dust with almond flour.
2. In a mixing bowl, combine all the ingredients, except the garnish, to form a dough.
3. Roll the dough into 20–24 small oblong shapes.
4. Place them on the prepared baking tray and, using a fork dipped in cacao powder, firmly press down on each biscuit. They should look like Nuttikrusts or old-style koffiekoekies, just healthier.
5. Garnish with coffee beans and hazelnuts or macadamia nuts if desired and bake for 7–10 minutes.
6. Remove from the oven and immediately drizzle with honey and dust with cacao powder or extra coffee grounds.
7. Allow to cool before storing in an airtight container in the fridge.

SERVINGS: 20—24 BISCUITS

If you are a coffee snob like me and appreciate a strong coffee taste, use ground coffee for a more intense flavour

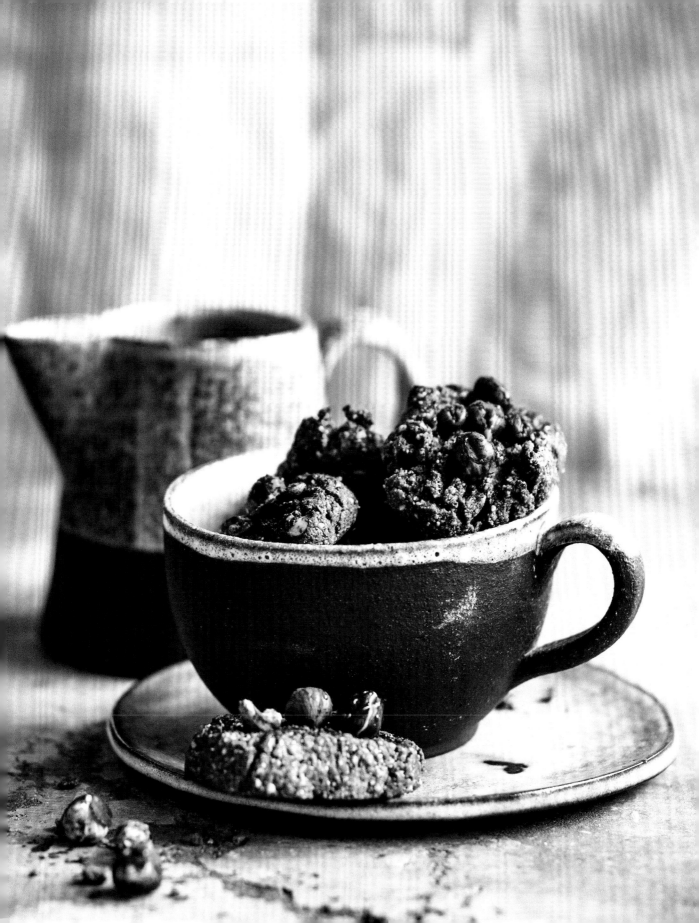

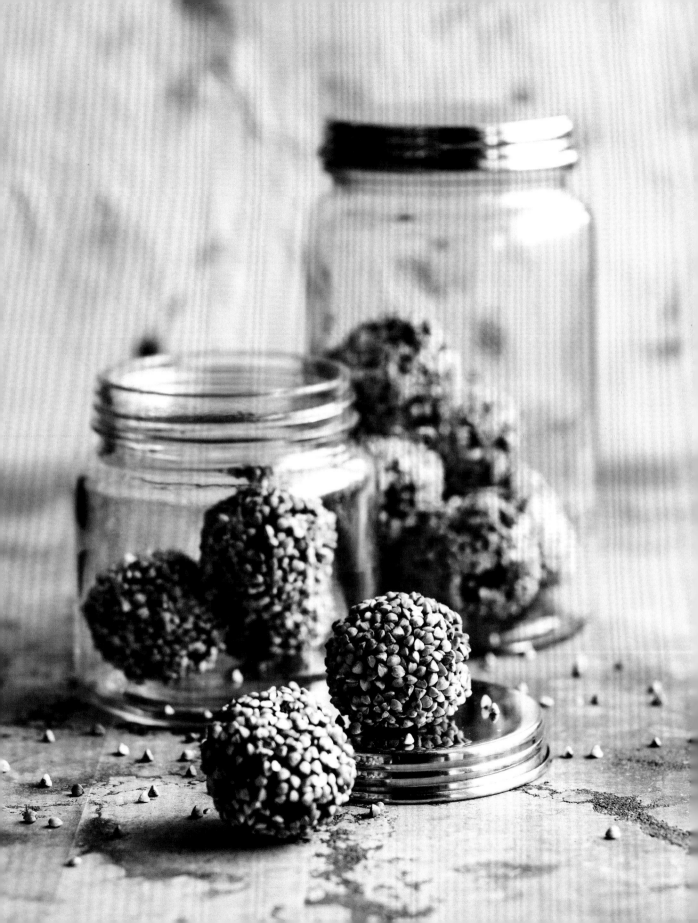

ROASTED BUCKWHEAT
BROWNIE BLISS BALLS

300 g pitted dates, chopped
300 g raisins
1 cup buckwheat
150 g almond flour
1 Tbsp caramel essence
4 heaped Tbsp raw cacao powder
1 tsp ground cinnamon
pinch of Oryx desert salt

Soak the dates and raisins in enough hot water to cover for 10–15 minutes. Drain and mash in a mixing bowl.

Spray a frying pan with non-stick cooking spray and roast the buckwheat over medium heat until light brown and toasted. It will smell like roasted nuts when ready. Set aside to cool.

Add the almond flour, caramel essence, cacao powder, cinnamon and salt to the mashed dates and raisins and mix well with your hands. To prevent the mixture sticking to your hands, spray your hands with non-stick cooking spray. Once they start to get sticky, wash your hands and spray again.

Place the mixture in the fridge to cool down. Once cooled, spray your hands with non-stick cooking spray and start rolling heaped teaspoons of the mixture into balls. Roll the balls in the roasted buckwheat.

Place the balls on a baking tray and refrigerate for at least 30 minutes until set.

Enjoy freshly made.

SERVINGS: 20 BLISS BALLS

Add 4-6 drops peppermint essence to the buckwheat while roasting for a crunchy peppermint variation xxx

Always a winner! Use this recipe to make muffins

CHOC CHIP BLONDIES

2 x 410 g cans chickpeas, drained and rinsed
6 Tbsp raw honey
100 g almond butter
1 tsp vanilla essence
2 tsp caramel essence
1 tsp bicarbonate of soda
50 g almond flour
1 tsp Oryx desert salt
2 large eggs
100 g dairy-free dark chocolate, chopped (I prefer Gayleen's Decadence)

1. Preheat the oven to 180 °C on thermo-fan. Line a 20 x 20 cm baking pan with baking paper and spray with non-stick cooking spray.
2. Place the chickpeas in the bowl of a food processor and blend until smooth. Add all the other ingredients, except the eggs and chocolate, and process on high for 3–5 minutes, scraping down the sides, until the mixture is smooth and well blended. (If you don't have a food processor, you can pulp the chickpeas with a blender, add the rest of the ingredients and beat with an electric beater for 2 minutes on high speed.)
3. Beat the eggs in a separate bowl until light and fluffy, then add to the chickpea mixture and beat for another 30 seconds to mix well. Fold in the chocolate chunks.
4. Spoon the mixture into the prepared baking pan, level it out and bake for 15–20 minutes. The edges will be crispy and firm to the touch, while the centre will remain moist and soft.
5. Allow to cool completely in the pan before cutting into squares and serving. The centre will firm up a bit while cooling, but will remain perfectly moist and soft.

NOTE: *These gluten-free soft and fudgy blondies are bursting with healthy flavour, are naturally sweetened and are the perfect dessert to sneak in some protein-packed chickpeas.*

SERVINGS: 12—16 BLONDIES

A handful of cranberries adds a powerful antioxidant punch!

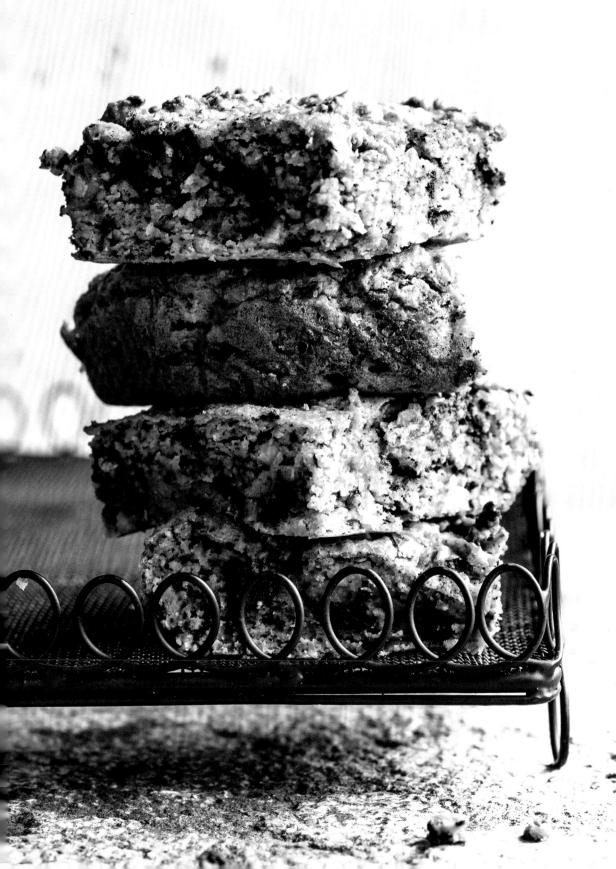

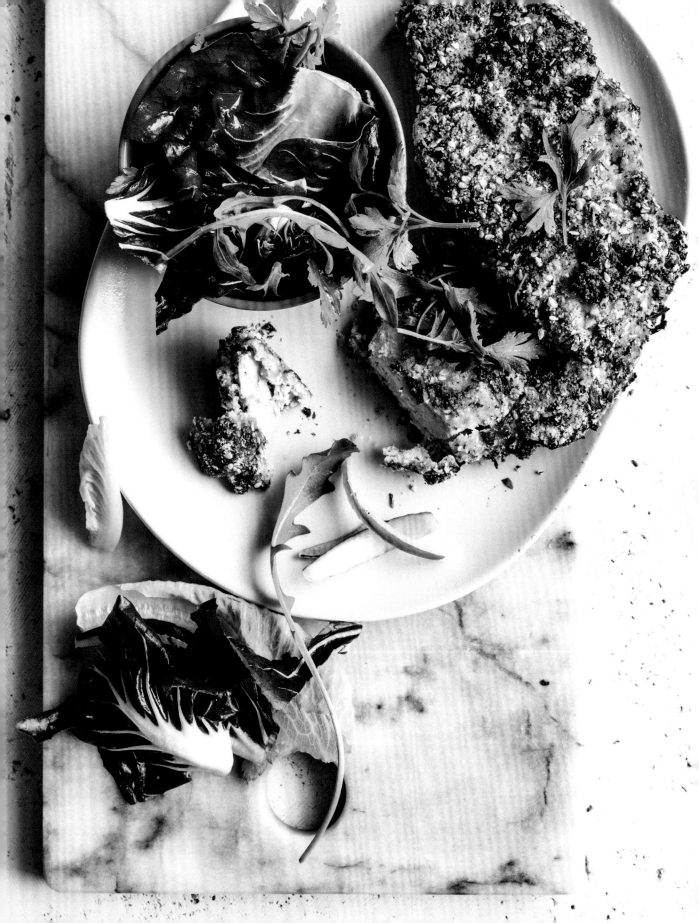

beloved classics

THROWBACK THURSDAY

This chapter is a throwback to my childhood. My love for cooking was born in our farmhouse kitchen, where I was always keen to help Mom and Dad whip up the next family breakfast, lunch or dinner. With a farmer for a dad and a landscaper for a mom, green fingers and lots of vegetables usually formed part of the meal planning for the day. These are all family favourites, with a healthy 'Izelle-approved' twist.

HEALTHY ALMOND FLOUR CHICKEN SCHNITZEL

1 cup almond flour
2 heaped Tbsp sesame seeds
1 heaped tsp crushed garlic
½ tsp fine Oryx desert salt
2 heaped tsp onion flakes
1 heaped tsp dried parsley
4 large eggs
4 large chicken fillets
3 Tbsp raw honey
4 tsp olive oil
pinch of paprika
handful of chopped fresh
Italian parsley

Preheat the oven to 200 °C. Line a baking tray with foil and spray with non-stick cooking spray.

Combine the almond flour, sesame seeds, garlic, salt, onion flakes and dried parsley in a shallow bowl.

Whisk the eggs in a separate bowl.

Place the chicken fillets on a flat surface and pat dry with paper towel. Place a sheet of cling film on top and gently tenderise the chicken using a mallet or rolling pin.

Seal both sides of the fillets with the honey.

Start by rolling the chicken fillets in the flour mixture so that it sticks to the honey, then dip them in the egg and roll in the flour again. Place on the prepared baking tray.

Bake for 20 minutes, then remove from the oven, drizzle with the oil and sprinkle with the paprika, and return to the oven for another 5 minutes.

Serve warm, garnished with the chopped fresh Italian parsley.

NOTE: _For a vegetarian option, cut a whole cauliflower into steaks and use the cauliflower steaks instead of chicken fillets._

SERVINGS: 4

One of Dad's favourites – just the healthy way

GINGER AND GARLIC BEEF STIR-FRY

250 g carrots, julienned
2 Tbsp sesame oil
1 medium or 2 small red
onions, sliced
1 heaped tsp crushed garlic
1 heaped tsp grated fresh ginger
600 g beef strips or cubes
5 Tbsp soy sauce
2 Tbsp sesame seeds
1 tsp ground black pepper
3 Tbsp raw honey
1 tsp Oryx desert salt
½ tsp chilli flakes
handful of chopped fresh
Italian parsley

1. Steam the carrots in a saucepan on the stove or in the microwave for 5 minutes. Set aside.
2. Heat the oil in a frying pan or wok over medium heat and fry the onion, garlic, ginger and beef until the meat is golden brown and cooked.
3. Combine the soy sauce, sesame seeds, black pepper, honey, salt and chilli flakes in a small bowl, and add to the pan or wok only once the meat is cooked. Simmer until most of the liquid has evaporated, then add the carrots and stir well.
4. Serve warm with rice or a side of your choice, garnished with the chopped fresh parsley.

NOTE: *This is also delicious served on a bed of greens as a salad. Just allow to cool completely.*

SERVINGS: 4

Ideal for the lunchbox the next day :-D

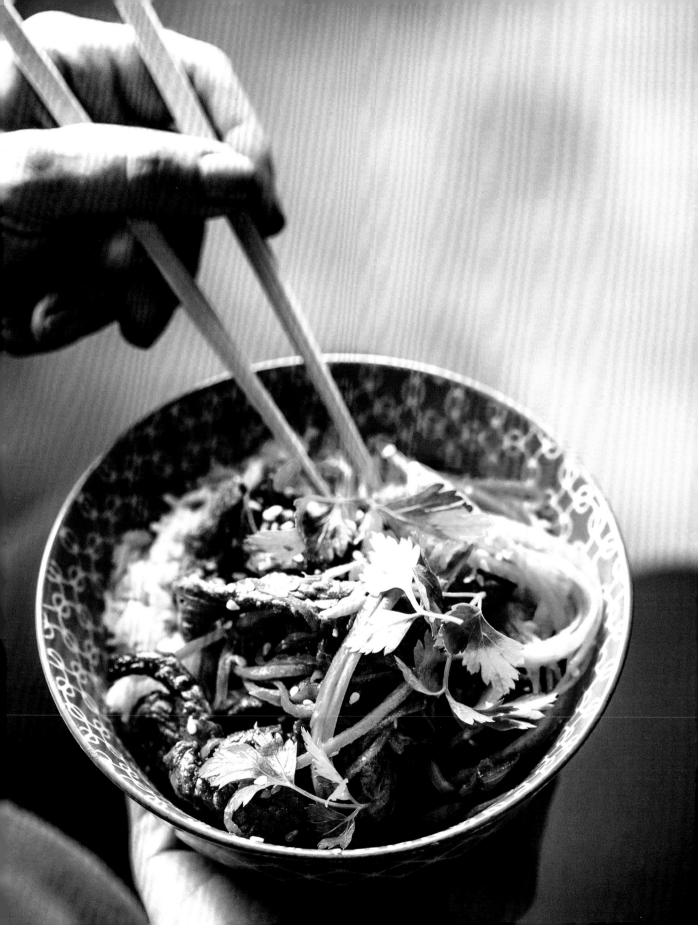

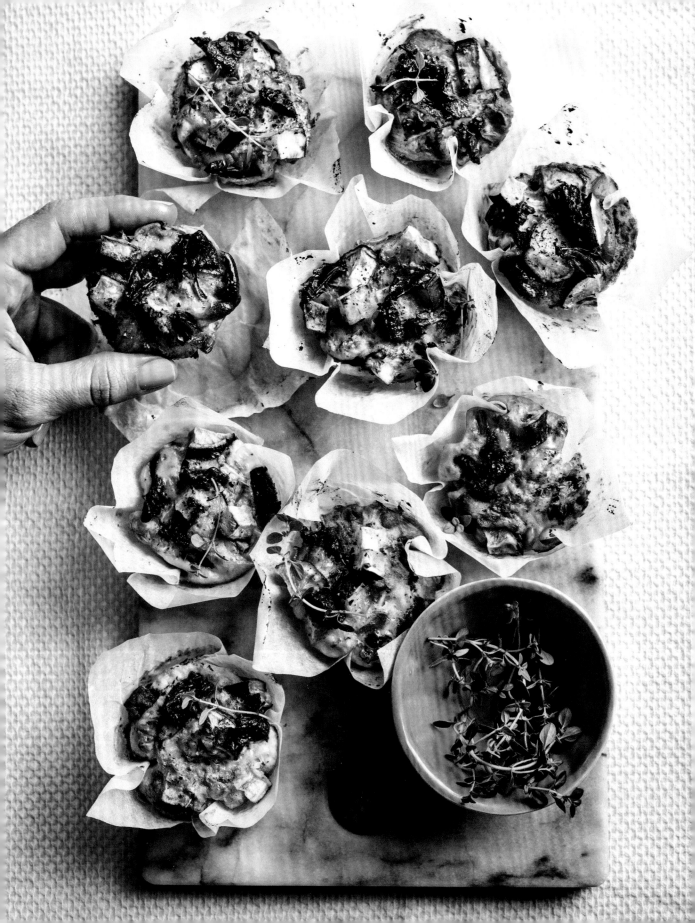

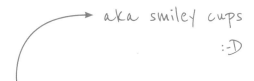
aka smiley cups
:-D

SUNDRIED TOMATO, BUTTERBEAN AND SWEET POTATO CUPS

1 Tbsp olive oil
1 large red onion, diced
1 tsp raw honey
pinch of Oryx desert salt
1 tsp paprika
1 x 410 g can butterbeans, drained
and rinsed
6 eggs
1 tsp dried thyme
300 g roasted or steamed sweet
potato chunks
50 g sundried tomatoes, chopped
(use kitchen scissors)
ground black pepper
fresh thyme for garnising

Preheat the oven to 200 °C and spray a muffin pan with non-stick cooking spray or line with paper cups.

Heat the oil in a saucepan and fry the onion until golden brown. Add the honey and salt and allow to caramelise. Stir in the paprika and butterbeans, and remove from the heat.

Whisk the eggs and thyme in a bowl.

Spoon the butterbean mixture into the muffin cups and top with the sweet potato and sundried tomatoes.

Divide the egg mixture between the muffin cups and season each with black pepper.

Bake for 25 minutes and serve garnished with fresh thyme.

SERVINGS: 12

Perfect for the lunchbox the next day and fantastic as a road-trip snack!

FAVOURITE!!!!!

OVEN-BAKED SALMON WITH CHILLI-LIME HONEY MARINADE

4 fresh salmon fillets
170 g small fresh asparagus spears
1 red bell pepper, deseeded and chopped into large pieces
1 orange or yellow bell pepper, deseeded and chopped into large pieces
1 green bell pepper, deseeded and chopped into large pieces
1 red onion, cut into wedges
pinch each of ground cumin, chilli flakes and Oryx desert salt
handful of chopped fresh parsley

CHILLI-LIME HONEY MARINADE

2 Tbsp olive oil
1 Tbsp water
1 Tbsp crushed garlic
1 tsp red chilli flakes
1 tsp ground cumin
2 tsp Oryx desert salt
2 Tbsp raw honey
1 tsp caramel essence
juice of 2 freshly squeezed limes

1. Preheat the oven to 200 °C and spray a baking tray with non-stick cooking spray.
2. Arrange the salmon fillets, asparagus, bell peppers and onion on the baking tray.
3. Mix all the marinade ingredients and pour about half over the fish and vegetables. Turn the fish and vegetables and pour over the rest of the marinade.
4. Sprinkle the fish with the cumin, chilli flakes and salt.
5. Bake for 8–10 minutes or until the fish is cooked to preference. If you prefer the vegetables to be softer, you can remove the fish fillets and bake the vegetables for another 10 minutes.
6. Garnish with the chopped fresh parsley before serving with basmati rice, salad or a side of your choice.

SERVINGS: 4

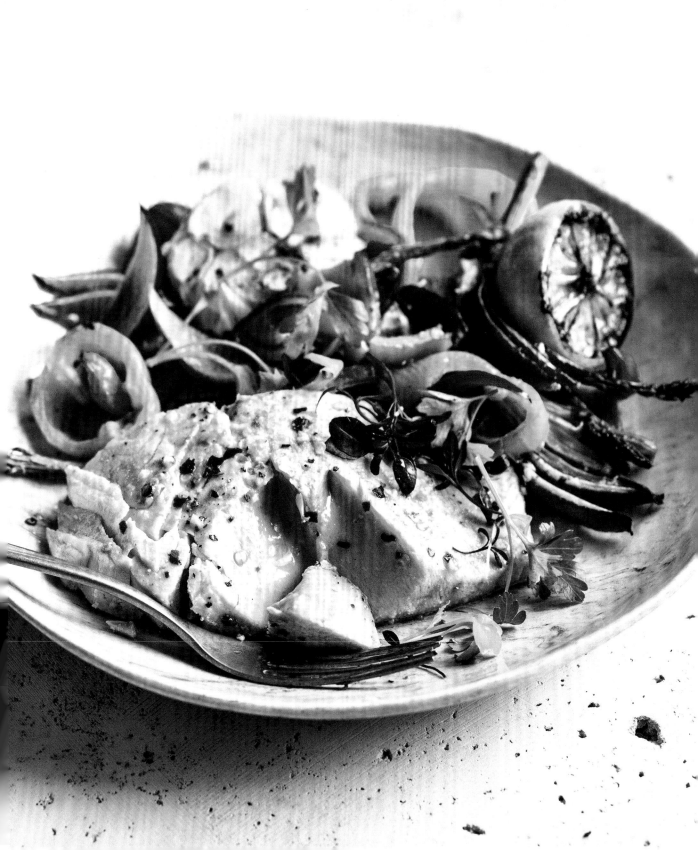

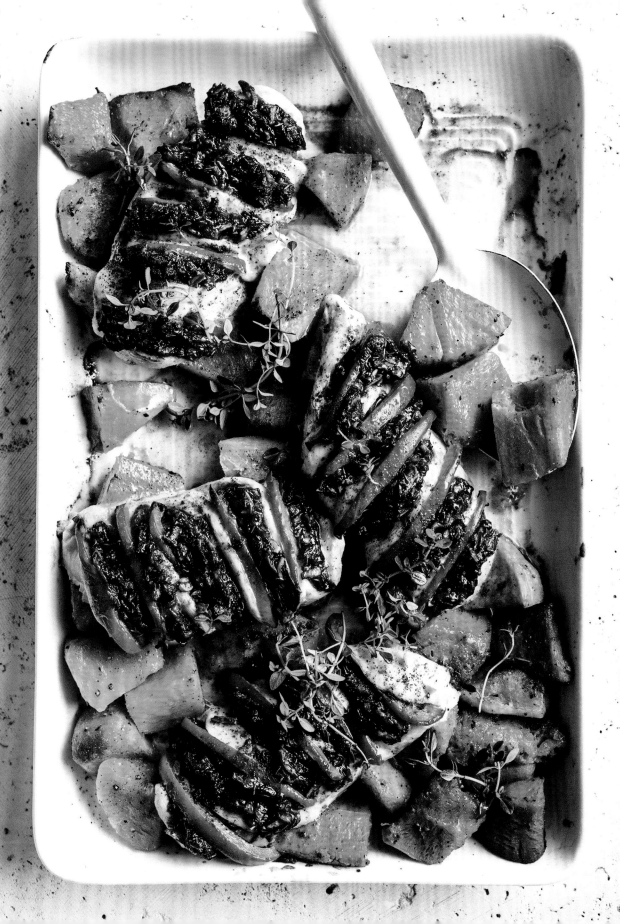

HASSEL 'HOFF' :-D

~~HASSELBACK~~ CHICKEN FILLET AND BUTTERNUT TRAY BAKE

1 kg pkt pre-cut butternut wedges
or chunks
2 Tbsp olive oil
2 Tbsp raw honey
Oryx desert salt, ground black
pepper and paprika
4 large chicken fillets (about
200 g each)
1 medium red bell pepper, deseeded
and cut into strips
fresh thyme for garnishing

SAUCE

1 medium red onion, diced
1 tsp Oryx desert salt
½ tsp ground black pepper
2 heaped Tbsp tomato paste
1 tsp paprika
2 Tbsp raw honey
1 heaped Tbsp onion flakes
1 tsp onion powder
1 Tbsp dried thyme
2 Tbsp water

Preheat the oven to 200 °C and spray a baking tray with non-stick cooking spray.

Cut a corner off the packet of butternut and microwave on high for 12 minutes.

Combine all the sauce ingredients.

Place the butternut in a large mixing bowl. Drizzle with the olive oil and honey, and season with salt, black pepper and paprika. Toss to coat and place on the greased baking tray.

Cut slits into the chicken fillets, about 1 cm apart and three-quarters of the way through. Tuck the red bell pepper strips into the slits and place the fillets on the baking tray on top of the butternut.

Scoop the sauce into the slits in the chicken with the bell pepper strips.

Bake for 20–25 minutes until the chicken is cooked through and the butternut is soft.

Garnish with fresh thyme before serving.

SERVINGS: 4

ROASTED SPAGHETTI SQUASH WITH CREAMY GARLIC SAUCE

1 large spaghetti squash (2–3 kg)
1 Tbsp olive oil
½ tsp Oryx desert salt
½ tsp ground black pepper
handful of chopped fresh
Italian parsley

CREAMY GARLIC SAUCE

1 x 410 g can butterbeans, drained
1 tsp olive oil
300 ml unsweetened almond milk
1 tsp crushed garlic
1 tsp onion powder
1 tsp Oryx desert salt
¼ tsp ground black pepper
1½ Tbsp raw honey

1. Preheat the oven to 200 °C and spray a baking tray with non-stick cooking spray.
2. Cut the squash into rounds and remove the seeds. Place the rounds on the baking tray and brush with the olive oil. Season with the salt and black pepper.
3. Bake for 30–40 minutes until tender and cooked.
4. In the meantime, make the sauce. Place the butterbeans in a blender or food processor and blend until smooth.
5. Spray a medium saucepan with non-stick cooking spray and add the butterbean purée along with the rest of the sauce ingredients. Bring to the boil over low heat, stirring regularly. Cook until the sauce has reached the desired thickness.
6. Use a fork to separate the strands of squash and transfer to a serving platter.
7. Pour over the sauce and garnish with the chopped fresh Italian parsley.

NOTE: *If you can't get spaghetti squash, you can use butternut or pumpkin 'spaghetti'. Simply arrange it on a baking tray, brush with olive oil and season with salt and black pepper, and bake for 10 minutes until cooked. Use forks to transfer it to your serving platter.*

SERVINGS: 4

Ideal for meat-free Mondays or add a protein of your choice – beef strips/chicken fillets/mince :-)

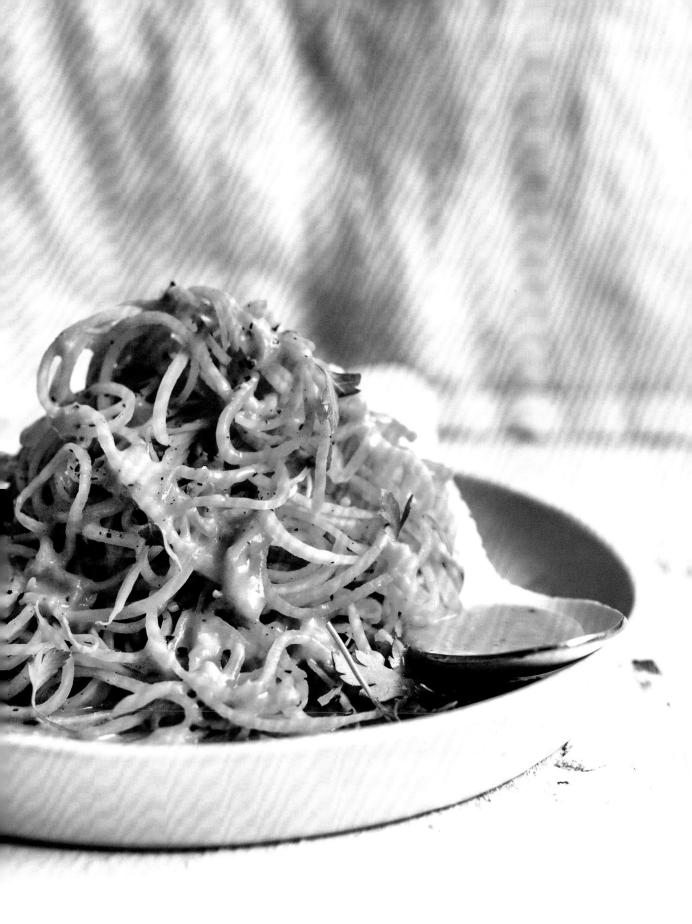

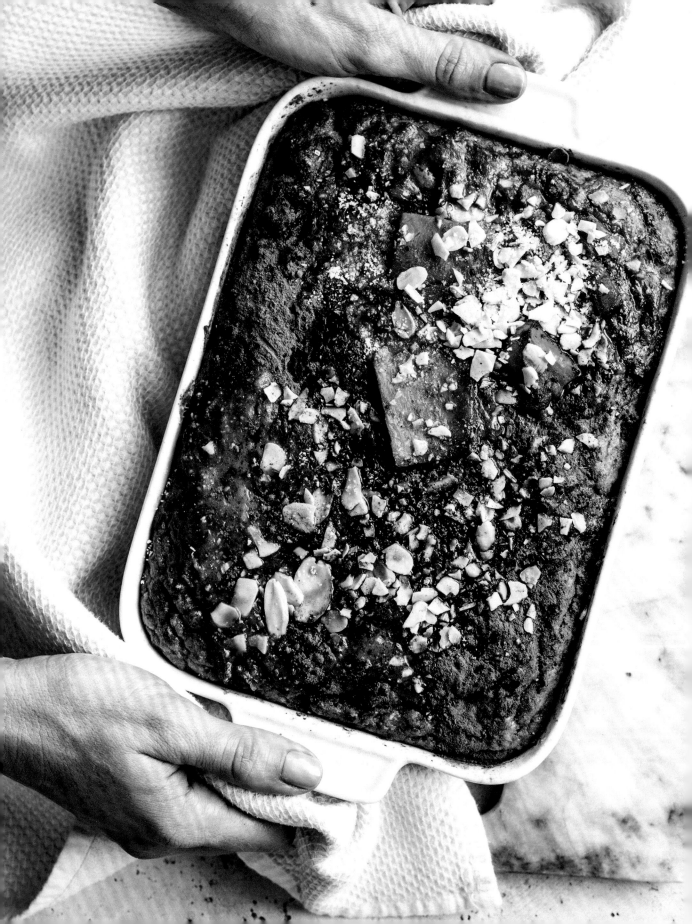

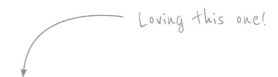
Loving this one!

'PUMPKIN' FRITTER BAKE

1 kg butternut mash
250 g almond flour
2 tsp Oryx desert salt
2 tsp caramel essence
1 tsp vanilla essence
2 tsp bicarbonate of soda
3 Tbsp raw honey
6 large eggs
butternut chunks for
garnishing (optional)
50 g diced almonds
¼ tsp ground cinnamon

SAUCE
150 g almond butter
1 tsp ground cinnamon
100 ml unsweetened almond milk
3 Tbsp raw honey
1 tsp Oryx desert salt
1 Tbsp vanilla essence

Preheat the oven to 200 °C and spray an ovenproof dish with non-stick cooking spray.
In a large mixing bowl, combine the butternut mash with the almond flour, salt, caramel essence, vanilla essence, bicarbonate of soda and honey.
Whisk the eggs in a separate bowl and then add to the butternut mixture. Mix well.
Pour the butternut batter into the greased dish and bake for 20 minutes. In the meantime, make the sauce by melting all the ingredients together in a saucepan.
After 20 minutes, remove the bake from the oven and pour over the sauce. Top with chunks of butternut if you like, sprinkle over the diced almonds and cinnamon and bake for another 20 minutes.
Serve warm as a side or as a dessert.

SERVINGS: 6–8

Literally tastes like pumpkin fritters in the form of a bake :-D

Impressive enough to impress the in-laws!

SWEET POTATO AND STRAWBERRY TART

CRUST

200 g dates
200 g almond flour
2 tsp caramel essence
½ tsp Oryx desert salt

FILLING

500 g sweet potato mash
100 g almond butter
1 Tbsp caramel essence
1 tsp vanilla essence
½ tsp Oryx desert salt
2 Tbsp raw honey
3 eggs

TOPPING

250 g fresh strawberries, chopped
1 tsp raw honey
1 tsp caramel essence
pinch of Oryx desert salt
handful of chopped fresh mint
½ tsp almond flour

1. Preheat the oven to 190 °C and spray a 23 cm pie dish with non-stick cooking spray.
2. To make the crust, soak the dates in enough hot water to cover until soft. Drain and mash.
3. Add the almond flour, caramel essence and salt and mix well to a crumb-like texture.
4. Spread the mixture on the bottom of the pie dish and press down firmly to form a pie crust on the base and up the sides.
5. To make the filling, mix the sweet potato mash, almond butter, caramel essence, vanilla essence, salt and honey in a mixing bowl. Whisk the eggs in a separate bowl until fluffy and then add to the mixture. Mix well and pour into the pie crust.
6. Bake for 15–20 minutes until the filling is set and the crust is dark golden brown. Allow to cool before topping.
7. Place the chopped strawberries in a mixing bowl along with the honey, caramel essence, salt and mint. Toss gently to coat and arrange on top of the cooled tart. Sprinkle with the almond flour and refrigerate until ready to serve.

SERVING: 1 LARGE TART

Top with nectarines, pineapples or even blueberries for variation :-D

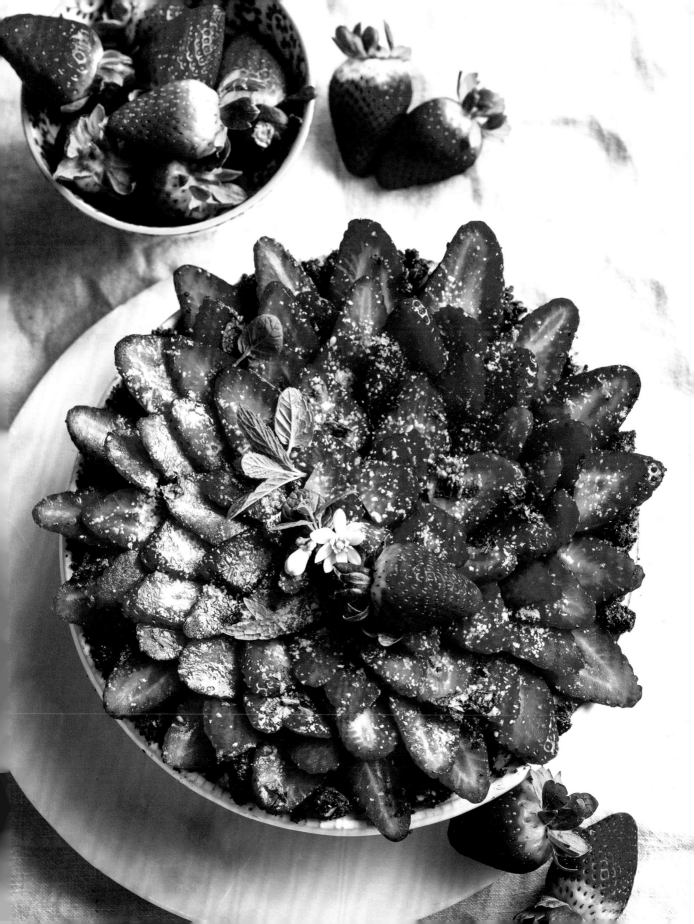

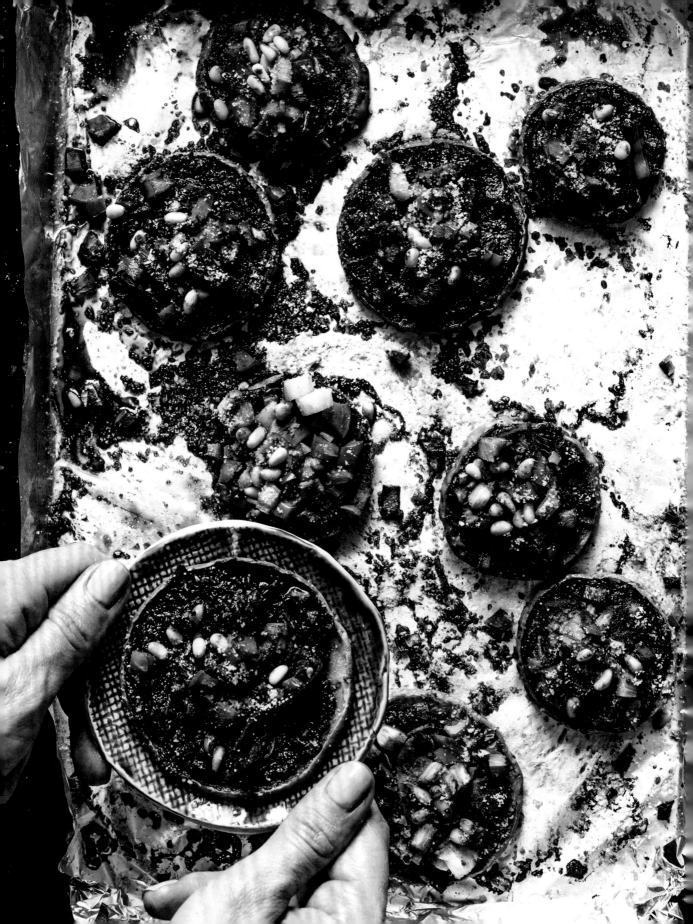

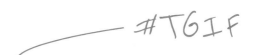
#TGIF

THANK GOODNESS IT'S FRIDAY!

Sides, sauces and snacks … Life is short, so enjoy party time around the snack platter! Sweet or savoury, I've got your back. And if you're having a braai, I just happen to have your back there too, because that's what friends are for.

MINI 'PIZZAS' *Yum!!!*

BASE
12–16 butternut or sweet potato rounds, cut 1 cm thick
olive oil
almond flour
Oryx desert salt
100 g baby spinach
6–8 tsp tomato paste

SAUCE
2 Tbsp soy sauce
2 Tbsp raw honey
1 heaped tsp crushed garlic
ground black pepper to taste

HAWAIIAN CHICKEN
pre-cooked chicken strips
diced fresh pineapple
diced red onion
diced mixed bell peppers
pine nuts

STEAK AND ONIONS
pre-cooked steak strips or mince
caramelised onions (fry diced onion in a bit of olive oil, with honey and salt until golden brown)
diced mixed bell peppers
pine nuts

Preheat the oven to 200 °C and spray a baking tray with non-stick cooking spray.

Place the butternut or sweet potato rounds on the tray and drizzle with a bit of olive oil, dust with almond flour and season with salt. Bake for 15 minutes.

Remove from the oven, turn over the rounds, and dress with more olive oil, almond flour and salt. Bake for another 10–15 minutes.

In the meantime, place the spinach in a bowl, cover with hot water and allow to stand for 5–10 minutes until wilted. Drain thoroughly, squeezing out as much moisture as possible.

To make the sauce, mix all the ingredients until the honey has dissolved in the soy sauce.

Smear each roasted butternut or sweet potato base with ½ tsp tomato paste and top with some wilted baby spinach, then add your choice of toppings and finish each off with a drizzle of the sauce.

Bake for 10–15 minutes or until the sauce starts to caramelise on top. These are best enjoyed warm.

NOTE: *Butternut contains about half the amount of carbohydrate than sweet potato, so if you feel like overindulging, go for the butternut for the 'pizza' bases. All topping options start with a basis of tomato paste and wilted baby spinach. After that, you can play around with toppings, but I've given you two of my favourite combinations.*

SERVINGS: 12–16

Perfect for a night in watching movies :-D

Use cauliflower florets for a vegetarian option

STICKY BBQ CHICKEN WINGS

8 chicken wings
1 Tbsp almond flour
chopped fresh thyme and lemon
wedges for garnishing

BASTING SAUCE
6 Tbsp olive oil
6 Tbsp raw honey
2 Tbsp water
1 Tbsp Oryx desert salt
1 heaped Tbsp sweet or
smoky paprika
1 Tbsp dried parsley

1. Preheat the oven to 200 °C. Line a baking tray with foil and spray with non-stick cooking spray.
2. Combine all the ingredients for the basting sauce in a mixing bowl.
3. Dip the chicken wings one at a time in the sauce, using your hands to make sure the whole wing is properly coated before placing it on the baking tray.
4. Dust the wings with the almond flour and bake for 20 minutes.
5. Remove from the oven and baste the wings with the leftover basting sauce. Switch the oven to grill and cook the wings for another 5 minutes.
6. Serve warm or cold, garnished with chopped fresh thyme and lemon wedges.

SERVINGS: 4

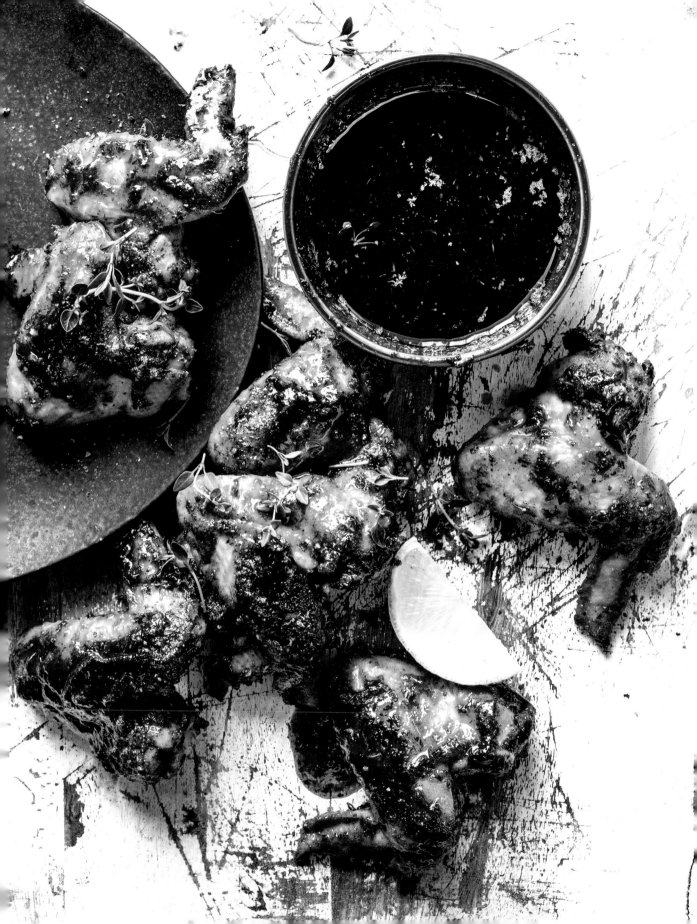

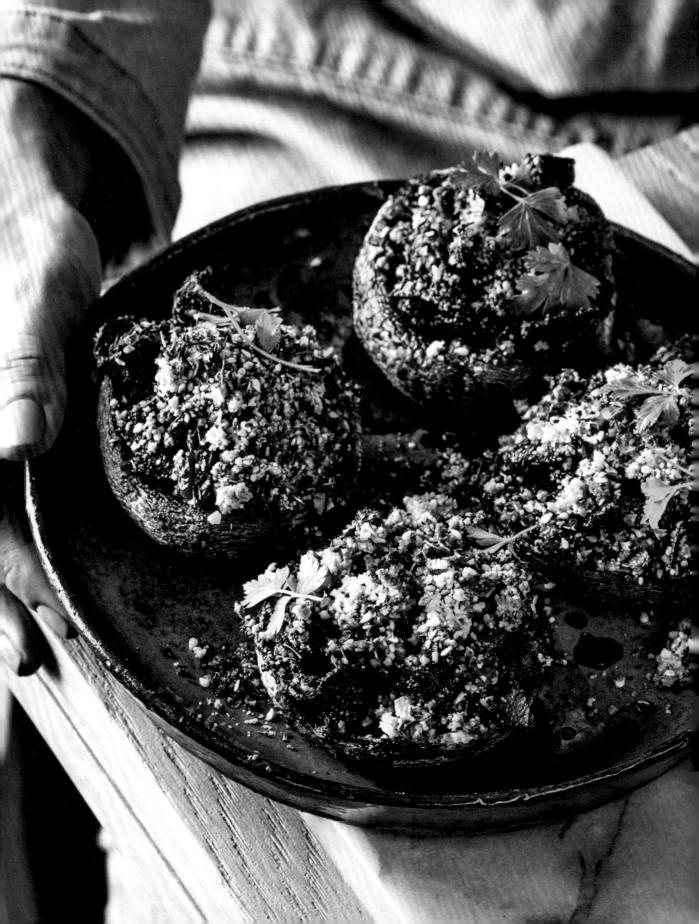

GRILLED PORTOBELLOS WITH BILTONG AND SUNDRIED TOMATOES

4 large portobello mushrooms
4 tsp olive oil
150 g shaved extra-lean moist biltong
120 g sundried tomatoes, chopped
1 heaped Tbsp almond flour
pinch of Oryx desert salt
½ tsp crushed garlic
1 heaped tsp sesame seeds
1 small red onion, chopped
¼ tsp dried parsley
¼ tsp ground black pepper
1 Tbsp raw honey
1 Tbsp soy sauce
chopped fresh Italian parsley for garnishing

Preheat the oven to 200 °C and spray a baking tray with non-stick cooking spray.

Place the mushrooms stem-side up on the tray and drizzle each with 1 tsp olive oil.

Top with biltong and then sundried tomatoes.

Using your fingertips, mix the almond flour, salt, garlic and sesame seeds to a large crumb-like texture.

Sprinkle the crumb on top of the mushrooms and finish each off with some chopped onion, dried parsley and black pepper.

Bake for 15 minutes, then remove from the oven and switch on the grill.

Mix the honey and soy sauce in a cup and drizzle over each mushroom.

Return to the oven to grill for 5 minutes.

Garnish with chopped fresh Italian parsley before serving.

SERVINGS: 4

Replace the biltong with 1 Tbsp cooked red quinoa per mushroom for a vegetarian option #winningatlife #Charlotte

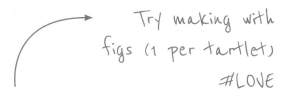

Try making with figs (1 per tartlet) #LOVE

CARAMELISED ONION AND GRAPE TARTLETS

2 Tbsp olive oil
1 red onion, diced
2 Tbsp raw honey
2 Tbsp balsamic vinegar
500 g sweet potato mash
1 cup almond flour, plus extra
for dusting
1 heaped tsp crushed garlic
2 heaped Tbsp sesame seeds
1 heaped tsp dried sage
1¼ tsp Oryx desert salt
2 eggs
350–400 g red globe grapes, halved
¼ tsp ground black pepper
30 g pine nuts
fresh sage for garnishing

1. Preheat the oven to 200 °C and spray a muffin pan with non-stick cooking spray or use muffin pan liners.
2. In a medium frying pan, heat 1 Tbsp of the oil and fry the onion until golden. Add the honey and balsamic vinegar and allow the onion to caramelise, but remove from the heat before the sauce gets completely sticky. Set aside.
3. In a mixing bowl, combine the sweet potato mash, almond flour, garlic, sesame seeds, dried sage and 1 tsp of the salt.
4. Whisk the eggs in a separate bowl until fluffy and then add to the sweet potato mixture. Stir well.
5. Scoop the sweet potato mixture into the muffin pan and create a tart shell in every cup by pressing the mixture into the base and sides. I prefer an uneven texture, so you don't need to smooth it out completely.
6. Place the grapes in a mixing bowl, add the black pepper and remaining oil and salt, and mix well.
7. Spoon the grapes into the potato-lined muffins cups, and top with the caramelised onion and pine nuts.
8. Bake for 25–30 minutes.
9. Allow to cool slightly before removing from the pan. Dust with almond flour and garnish with fresh sage before serving.

SERVINGS: 12—16

You'll knock everyone's socks off when you arrive at a kitchen tea with these crowd-pleasers

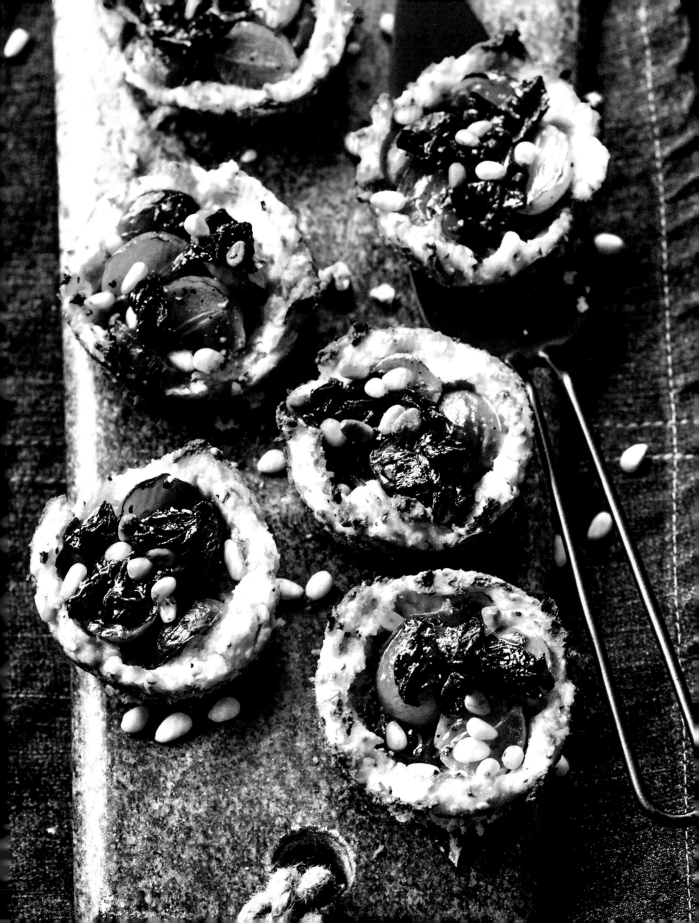

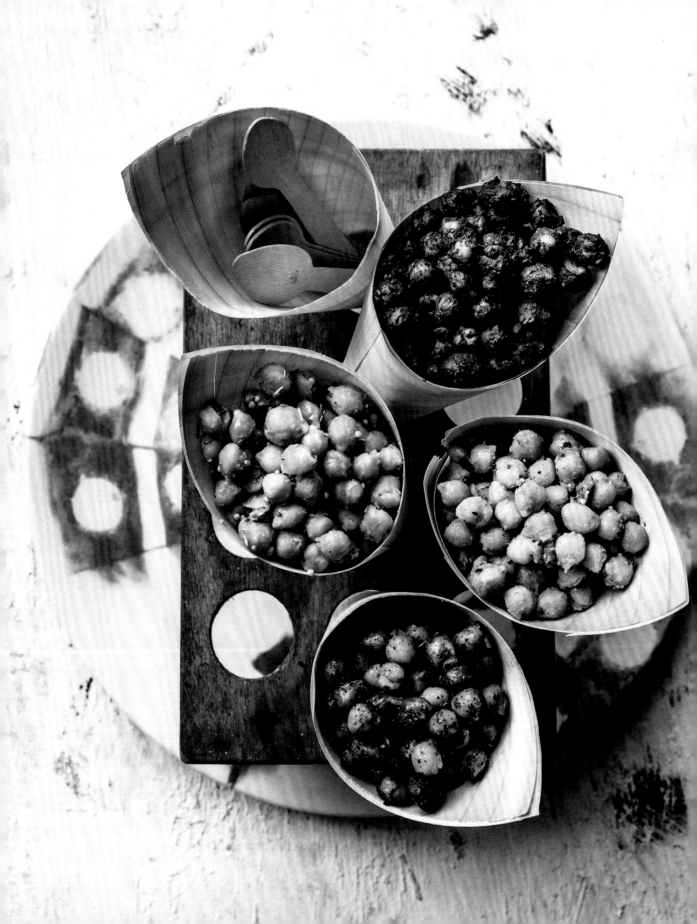

ROASTED CHICKPEAS 4 WAYS

2 x 410 g cans chickpeas, drained
2 Tbsp olive oil
2 Tbsp raw honey

CINNAMON CHOCOLATE

2 tsp caramel essence
1 tsp Oryx desert salt
¼ cup raw cacao powder
2 tsp ground cinnamon
1 tsp ground nutmeg
2 Tbsp almond flour

TURMERIC AND BLACK PEPPER

2 tsp onion powder
2 tsp ground turmeric
2 tsp ground black pepper
2½ tsp Oryx desert salt (reserve
½ tsp for sprinkling over
once cooked)

HONEY-MUSTARD AND ROSEMARY

2 tsp onion powder
2 tsp mustard powder
2 tsp mustard seeds
2 tsp dried rosemary
2½ tsp Oryx desert salt (reserve
½ tsp for sprinkling over
once cooked)

BBQ

2 heaped tsp paprika
1 tsp ground black pepper
2 tsp dried parsley
2½ tsp Oryx desert salt (reserve
½ tsp for sprinkling over
once cooked)

Preheat the oven to 190 °C and spray a baking tray with non-stick cooking spray.

Rinse the chickpeas, pat dry with paper towel and place in a mixing bowl.

Drizzle the chickpeas with the olive oil and honey and add the flavouring of your choice.

Mix well until all the chickpeas are evenly coated.

Bake for 35–40 minutes, stirring occasionally, until crisp.

NOTE: *Best served straight from the oven.*

SERVINGS: 4–6

Snack away, the healthy way!

CANDIED BILTONG CLUSTERS

2 Tbsp caramel essence
3 Tbsp olive oil
3 Tbsp raw honey
2 Tbsp water
1 tsp Oryx desert salt
½ tsp ground cinnamon
¼ tsp cayenne pepper
300 g extra-lean moist biltong
100 g pecan nuts, crushed
2 heaped Tbsp almond flour

1. Preheat the oven to 200 °C and line a baking tray with baking paper.
2. In a medium mixing bowl, combine the caramel essence, oil, honey, water, salt, cinnamon and cayenne pepper.
3. Add the biltong and pecan nuts and mix with your hands until well coated.
4. Spread evenly on the baking tray, sprinkle with the almond flour and bake for 20–25 minutes until candied and crisp, tossing halfway.

NOTE: *Serve with dates on the side for an extra sweet twist.*

SERVINGS: 4–6

Someone is going to lick the bowl, guaranteed! :-D

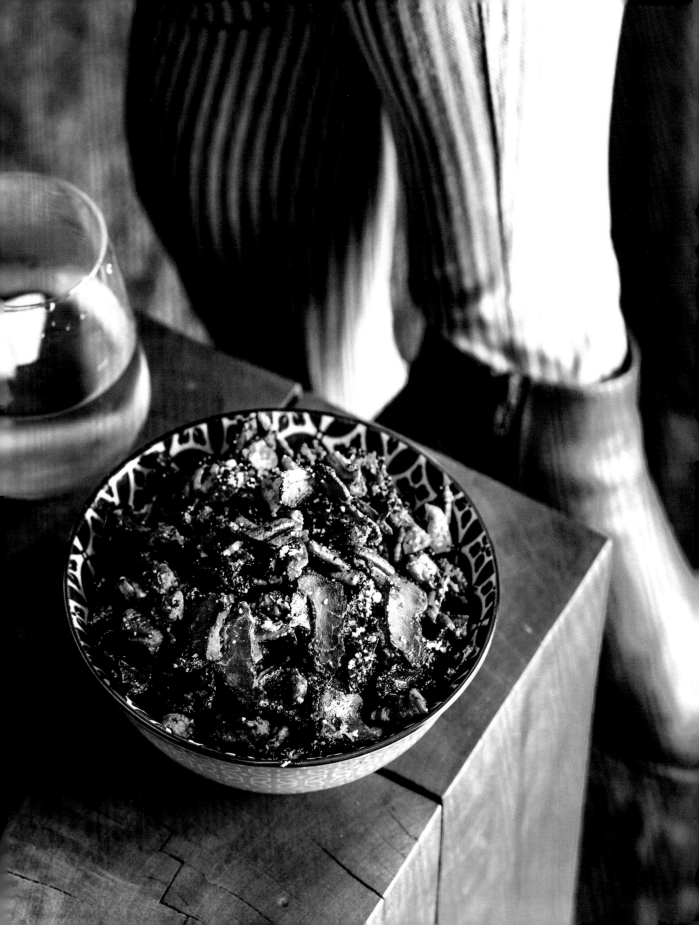

BAKED BUTTERBEAN DIP WITH ALMOND CRUST

3 Tbsp olive oil
2 medium red onions, diced
1 tsp crushed garlic
1 tsp dried rosemary
1 tsp dried thyme
3 Tbsp raw honey
2 tsp Oryx desert salt
½ tsp ground black pepper
2 Tbsp tahini
½ tsp garlic powder
2 x 410 g cans butterbeans, drained,
rinsed and mashed
chopped fresh thyme for garnishing

ALMOND CRUST
60 g almond flour
1 tsp garlic flakes
1 tsp onion powder
1 tsp Oryx desert salt
2 tsp dried parsley
2 tsp olive oil

1. Preheat the oven to 200 °C and spray a small baking dish with non-stick cooking spray.
2. Heat the oil in a frying pan and fry the onions, crushed garlic, rosemary and thyme until golden brown. Add 2 Tbsp of the honey and fry until the onions are caramelised. Season with 1 tsp of the salt and the black pepper.
3. In a mixing bowl, mix the tahini, garlic powder, remaining salt, remaining honey and mashed butterbeans and add to the onions in the pan. Stir and then transfer to the greased baking dish. Spread out evenly.
4. Mix the ingredients for the almond crust and spread over the butterbean dip.
5. Bake for 8–10 minutes or until the crust is crispy and golden brown.
6. Allow to cool and then refrigerate until properly set.
7. Garnish with chopped fresh thyme and serve with biltong, droëwors and salted crackers of your choice.

SERVINGS: 4—6

A real party starter :-D

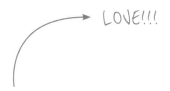
LOVE!!!

CINNAMON SWEET POTATO CHIPS WITH SALTED CARAMEL DATE DIPPING SAUCE

1 kg whole sweet potatoes, washed
2 Tbsp olive oil
2 Tbsp raw honey
½ tsp Oryx desert salt
1 tsp ground cinnamon

SALTED CARAMEL DATE DIPPING SAUCE

1 cup unsweetened almond milk
300 g fresh pitted Medjool dates
1 cup hot water
2 tsp caramel essence
1 tsp vanilla essence
1 tsp Oryx desert salt
¼ tsp ground cinnamon
¼ tsp ground nutmeg
1 heaped tsp almond butter

Preheat the oven to 200 °C. Line a baking tray with foil and spray with non-stick cooking spray.

Thinly slice the unpeeled sweet potatoes into round chips and place in a large mixing bowl. You want them thin like potato crisps, so use a mandoline slicer.

Combine the olive oil, honey, salt and cinnamon and pour this over the sweet potato chips. Mix well until all the chips are evenly coated.

Place on the prepared baking tray and bake for 30–40 minutes until crisp.

To make the dipping sauce, spray a large saucepan with non-stick cooking spray.

Add the almond milk, dates, hot water, caramel essence, vanilla essence, salt, cinnamon and nutmeg.

Cook until the dates are soft and most of the liquid has evaporated.

Remove from the heat, mash until smooth and stir in the almond butter.

Serve the sweet potato chips with the dipping sauce on the side.

NOTE: *Don't scrub the sweet potatoes, as the skin contains most of the fibre. Rather just soak and wash them.*

SERVINGS: 4–6

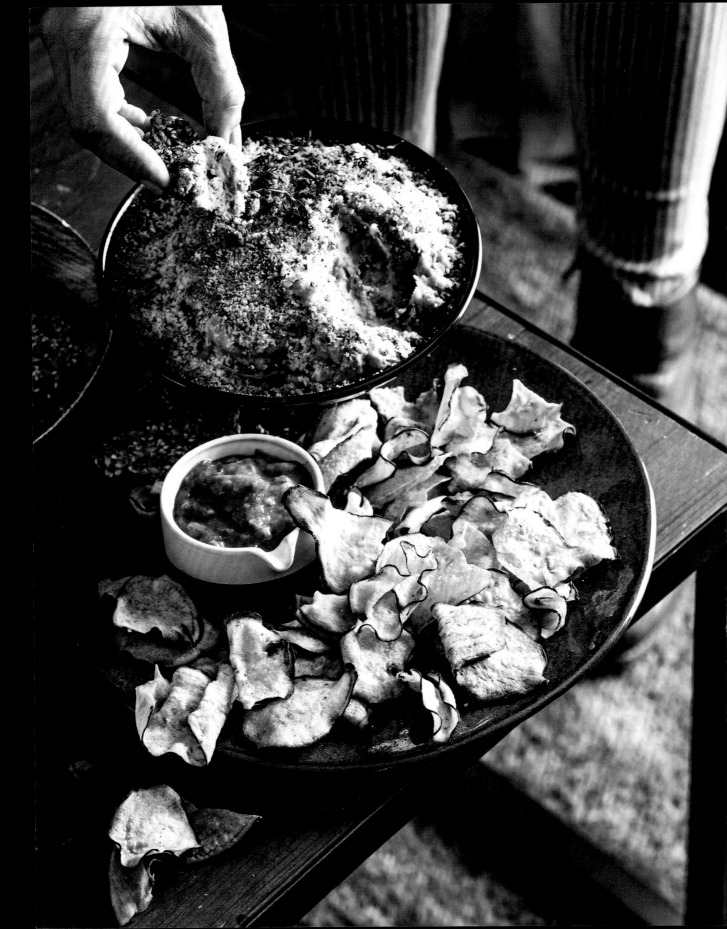

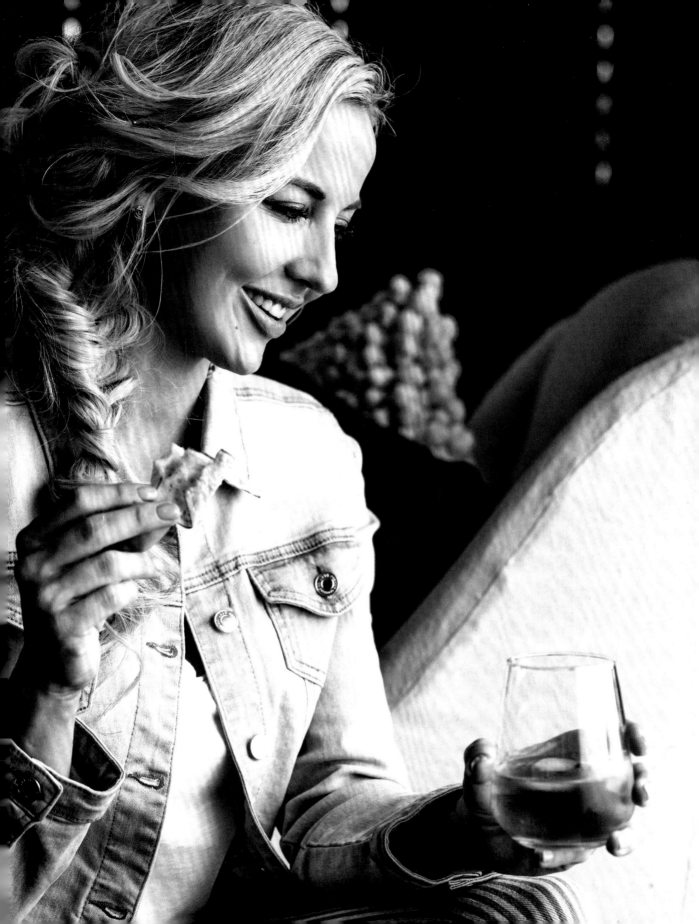

Love is ... toasted dessert :-D

DESSERT BRAAI BREAD

3 tsp olive oil
3 eggs
Oryx desert salt
1 tsp caramel essence
1 tsp raw cacao powder (optional)
2 slices bread of your choice (I prefer
100% rye)
2 tsp almond butter
2 tsp raw honey, plus extra
for drizzling
80 g sliced banana
a few sliced fresh strawberries
(optional)
1 marshmallow, cut up (optional, for
a naughty add-on)
¼ tsp ground cinnamon
2 tsp flaked almonds

1. Spray a frying pan with non-stick cooking spray and heat 1 tsp of the olive oil.
2. In a mixing bowl, beat the eggs, ½ tsp salt and caramel essence until fluffy. If you are making chocolate toast, add the cacao powder to the egg mixture now.
3. Soak the bread in the egg, transfer to the pan and cook on both sides until almost crispy.
4. Allow to cool slightly before buttering each slice with the almond butter followed by the honey and a pinch of salt. Top one slice with the banana, strawberries (if using), marshmallow (if using), cinnamon and flaked almonds and use the other slice to close the sandwich.
5. Place the sandwich in a braai grid and brush both sides lightly with the remaining olive oil. Braai until toasted and nice and crispy. Drizzle with honey and serve immediately.

SERVINGS: 1

Can be made in a sandwich press

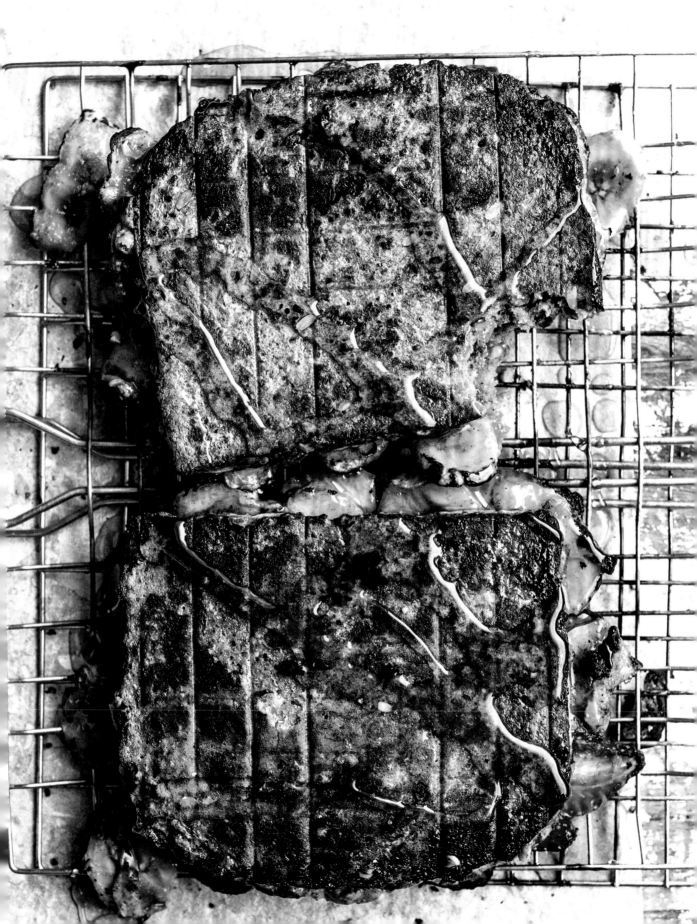

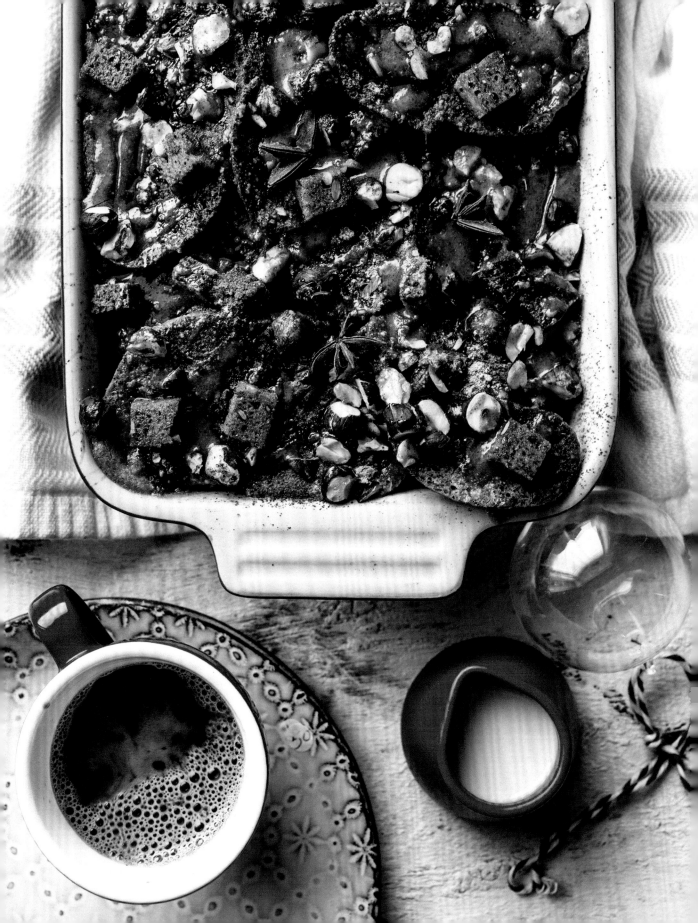

FOR THE LOVE OF FAMILY

Nothing beats spending festive and special occasions with family and friends. Turn that FOMO (fear of missing out) into YOLO (you only live once) and make every second count! Time and health are the two things that money can't buy, so spend some quality time with those who matter by sharing food made with love.

GINGERBREAD FRENCH TOAST BREAKFAST BAKE

3 eggs
150 ml unsweetened almond milk
6 Tbsp raw honey, plus extra for drizzling
1 tsp ground cinnamon, plus extra for sprinkling
1 tsp ground ginger, plus extra for sprinkling
½ tsp ground allspice
½ tsp ground nutmeg
½ tsp ground cloves
½ tsp Oryx desert salt
1.2 kg 100% rye bread, sliced 1 cm thick
handful of whole or chopped hazelnuts

SAUCE
150 g almond butter
150 ml unsweetened almond milk
2 tsp caramel essence
½ tsp Oryx desert salt
3 Tbsp raw honey

Spray a rectangular 20 x 30 cm baking dish with non-stick cooking spray. In a mixing bowl, whisk the eggs and then add the almond milk, honey and all the spices. Mix well.

Pour just enough egg mixture into the baking dish to cover the bottom and form a base.

Place a layer of bread in the bottom of the dish and pour over some more of the egg mixture. Repeat the layers until the dish is full, ending with egg mixture. Any bread cut-offs can be sliced into small crouton-like cubes to be sprinkled over the top.

Mix all the sauce ingredients and pour over the eggy bread. Sprinkle with cinnamon, ginger, hazelnuts and 'croutons' and refrigerate overnight.

The next morning, preheat the oven to 180 °C. Drizzle the dish with honey and bake for 25–30 minutes. You can bake it straight from the fridge. Serve warm with cups of coffee.

NOTE: *You can use a different type of bread, but I find the spices in rye bread add to the flavour.*

SERVINGS: 6–8

Perfect for Christmas morning; literally tastes like love on a plate!

OSTRICH FILLET WITH BALSAMIC CRANBERRY GLAZE

500 g ostrich fillet
olive oil for frying
fresh thyme for garnishing

BALSAMIC CRANBERRY GLAZE

3 Tbsp olive oil
3 Tbsp balsamic vinegar
1 tsp Oryx desert salt
½ tsp ground black pepper
1 heaped tsp paprika
1 Tbsp raw honey
1 tsp caramel essence
handful of dried cranberries

1. Combine all the glaze ingredients and mix well until the honey has dissolved.
2. Baste the fillet on both sides with some of the glaze.
3. Heat a drizzle of olive oil in a frying pan and fry the fillet for 4 minutes on each side for medium-rare.
4. Remove the meat from the pan and set aside to rest.
5. Pour the leftover glaze into the pan and simmer until thickened. Place the fillets back in the pan and baste with the glaze.
6. Garnish with fresh thyme before serving.

SERVINGS: 3—4

*Perfect with beef fillet too!
Ideal to serve with oven-roasted sweet
potato wedges or beetroot crisps*

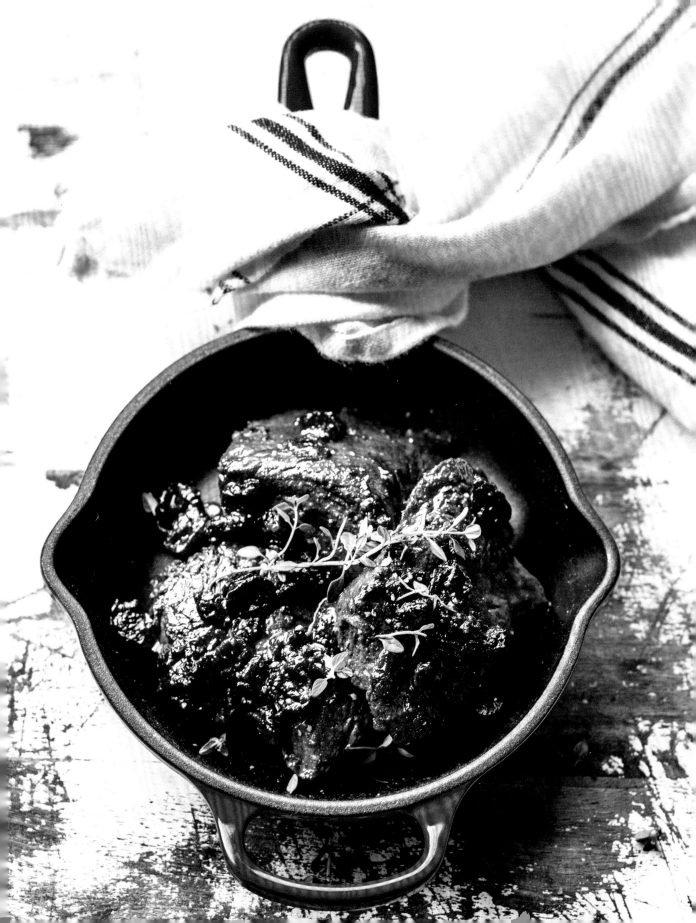

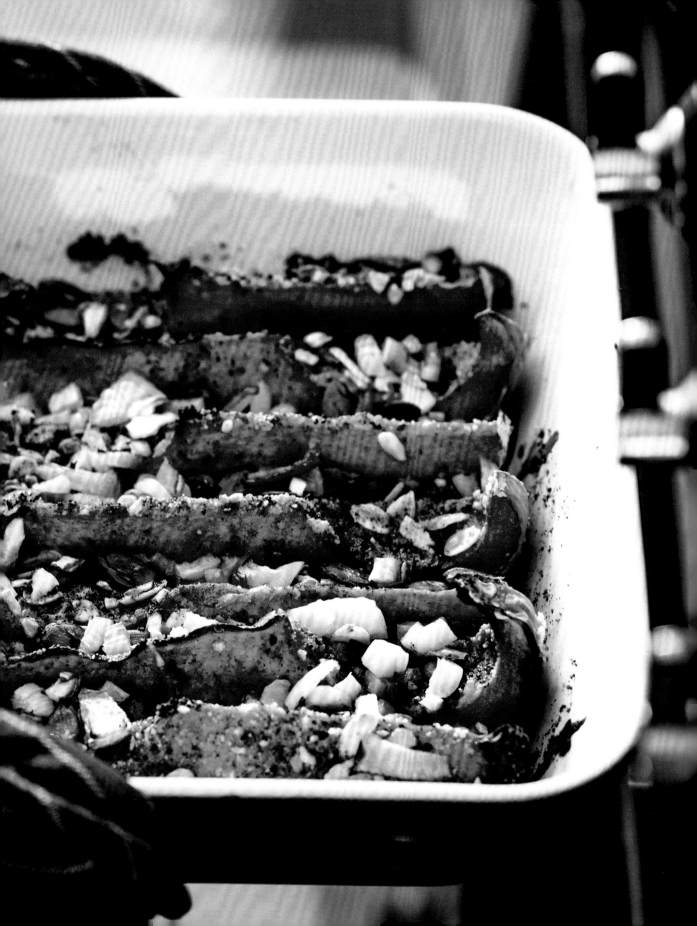

OVEN-ROASTED BUTTERNUT WEDGES

2 medium whole butternuts
8 tsp olive oil (1 tsp per wedge)
¼ tsp Oryx desert salt
50 g almond flour
1 tsp caramel essence
1 Tbsp raw honey
20 g diced almonds
¼ tsp ground black pepper
¼ tsp paprika
4 small red onions, diced
20 g pumpkin seeds
chopped fresh rosemary
for garnishing

Preheat the oven to 200 °C. Line a baking tray with foil and spray with non-stick cooking spray.

Cut each butternut into quarters and remove the seeds.

Arrange the butternut wedges on the baking tray and drizzle each with 1 tsp olive oil. Dress with the salt, almond flour, caramel essence and honey. Finish off with the diced almonds and black pepper.

Roast for 30 minutes, then remove from the oven and sprinkle over the paprika, onions and pumpkin seeds.

Roast for another 15 minutes and garnish with chopped fresh rosemary before serving.

SERVINGS: 4

Serve with chicken, lamb, beef or even quinoa :-D

Braai Day show-stopper all the way :-D

LAMB AND FIG SKEWERS WITH MINTY APRICOT GLAZE

600 g lamb, cut into chunky cubes
12 spring onions, cut into
4 cm pieces
6 fresh figs, halved
1 Tbsp olive oil
fresh mint for garnishing

MINTY APRICOT GLAZE

200 g dried apricots, chopped
2 cups hot water
2 Tbsp raw honey
zest of 1 lemon
2 Tbsp red wine vinegar
1 tsp chilli flakes
1 tsp crushed garlic
1 tsp Oryx desert salt
handful of chopped fresh mint

1. If using wooden or bamboo skewers, soak them in water for at least 30 minutes – this will prevent the glaze from sticking and burning during cooking.
2. Thread the skewers starting with a piece of lamb, followed by spring onion, half a fig and spring onion again. Repeat.
3. Heat the olive oil in a frying pan and cook the skewers for about 3 minutes on each side. Alternatively, drizzle the skewers with the olive oil and cook on the braai.
4. In the meantime, combine all the glaze ingredients in a saucepan. Bring to a simmer and allow some of the liquid to evaporate until you get a relatively thick sauce.
5. Once the skewers are cooked, pour over some of the glaze and cook for a further 30 seconds.
6. Garnish with fresh mint and serve immediately with the leftover glaze on the side.

SERVINGS: 6

Make it fresh and you WILL impress!

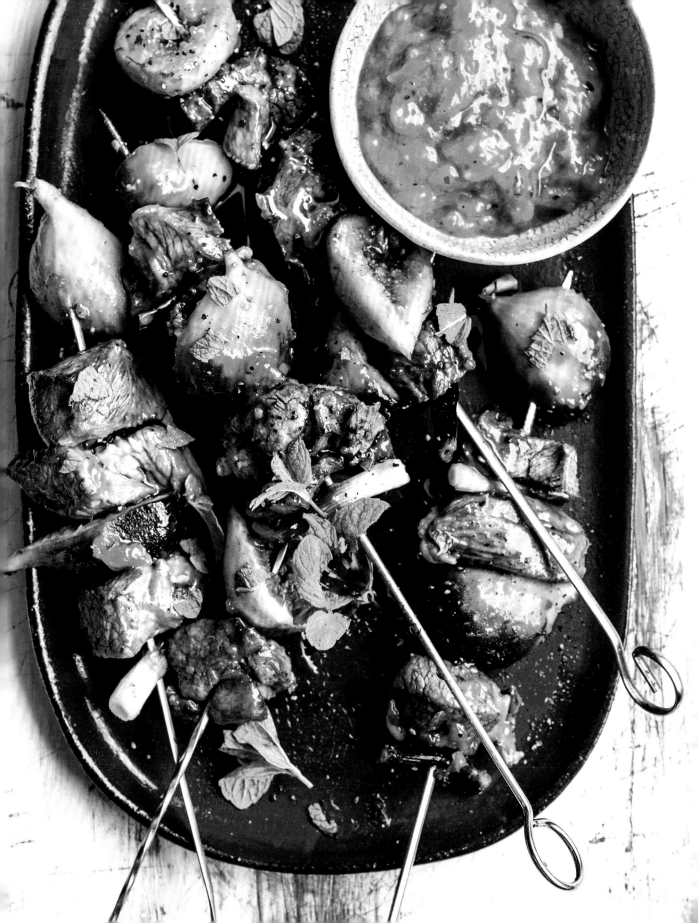

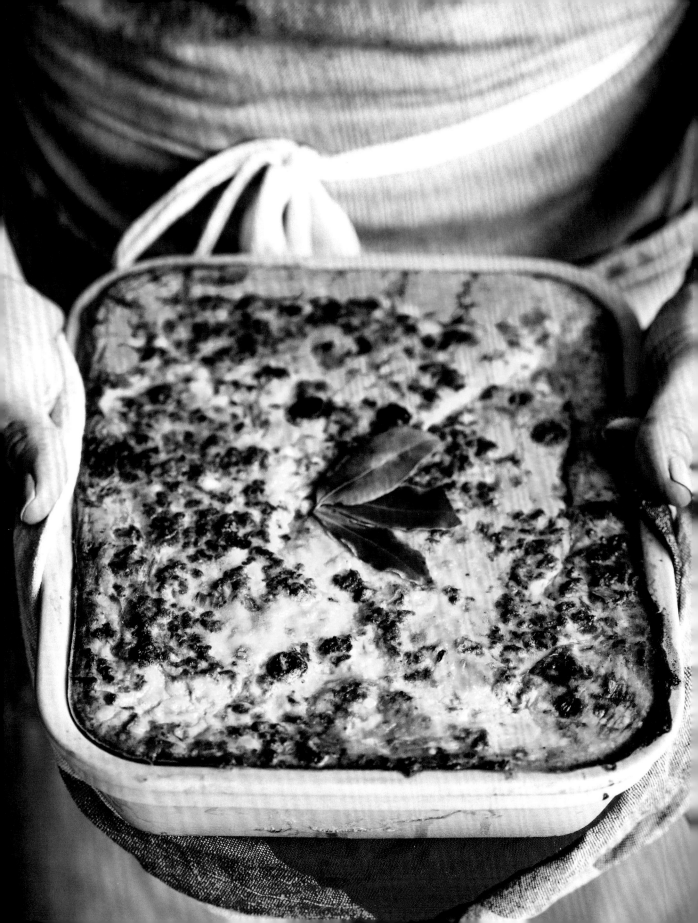

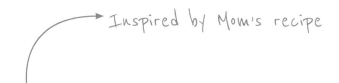

Inspired by Mom's recipe

HEALTHY BOBOTIE

2 tsp olive oil
1 red onion, chopped
2 tsp crushed garlic
1.25 kg extra-lean beef mince
¼ cup lemon juice
¼ cup raw honey
1 tsp ground cloves
1 Tbsp Oryx desert salt
1 Tbsp curry powder
2 tsp ground turmeric
5 bay leaves, finely crushed
100 g raisins
2 eggs, whisked
6 eggs
1 cup unsweetened almond milk
3 whole bay leaves

Preheat the oven to 180 °C and spray an ovenproof dish with non-stick cooking spray.

Heat the olive oil in a big frying pan and fry the onion and garlic until golden brown.

Add the mince and fry until browned, then remove the pan from the heat.

Add the lemon juice, honey, spices, raisins and whisked eggs to the mince. Stir well.

Place the mince mixture in the greased dish and compact with a large spoon.

Beat the 6 eggs and almond milk in a mixing bowl and pour over the mince.

Finish off with the whole bay leaves and bake for 40 minutes or until the egg is set.

NOTE: *Serve with yellow rice and freshly sliced banana. Homemade chutney rounds it off perfectly.*

SERVINGS: 6–8

One of my all-time favourites!!!

ASIAN-STYLE CHICKEN

2 large spring onions, diced
1 small red bell pepper, deseeded
and diced
1 small yellow bell pepper, deseeded
and diced
1 small green bell pepper, deseeded
and diced
5–6 chicken fillets or 9 drumsticks
and thighs
2 Tbsp olive oil
¼ cup hot water
chopped fresh coriander and spring
onion for garnishing

SAUCE
juice of 1 lime
¼ cup soy sauce
2 Tbsp raw honey
2 Tbsp olive oil
½ tsp crushed garlic
1 heaped Tbsp sesame seeds
½ tsp Oryx desert salt
½ tsp ground black pepper
½ tsp crushed fresh ginger (optional)
handful of chopped fresh coriander

1. Preheat the oven to 200 °C and spray an ovenproof dish with non-stick cooking spray.
2. Spread the diced spring onions and bell peppers on the base of the greased dish.
3. Brush the chicken pieces with the olive oil and place on top of the onions and peppers.
4. Pour the hot water around the chicken.
5. Mix the sauce ingredients in a small bowl and pour over the chicken pieces.
6. Cover with foil and bake for 30 minutes, then remove the foil and bake uncovered for a further 15 minutes, occasionally basting the chicken pieces with the sauce in the dish.
7. Garnish with chopped fresh coriander and spring onion before serving.

NOTE: *Ideal with a side salad, roast vegetables and basmati rice or quinoa, and long-stem broccoli florets, of course.*

SERVINGS: 4–6

Inspired by another of Mom's recipes

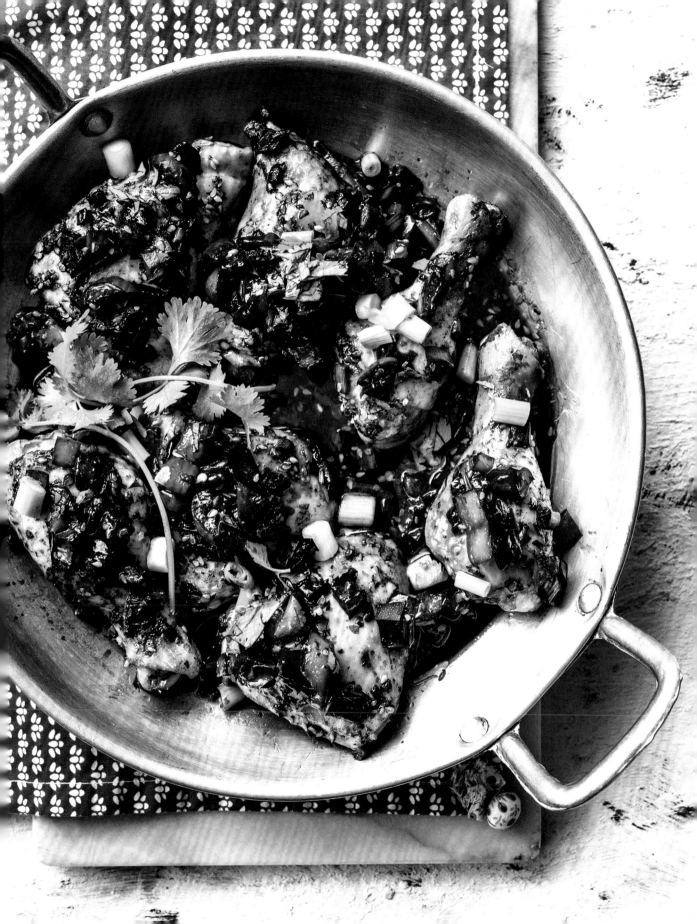

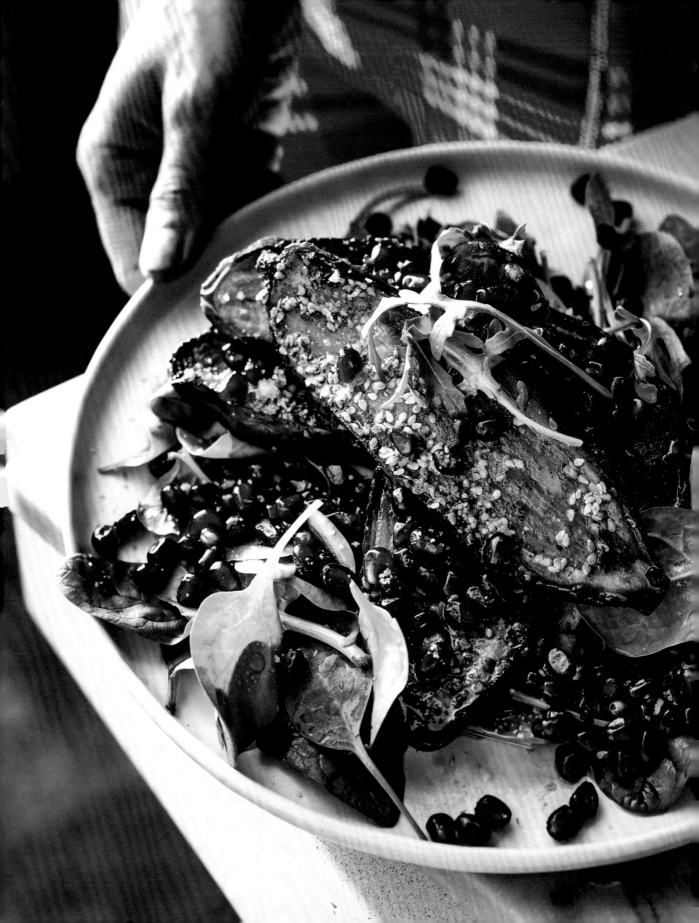

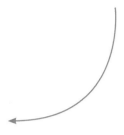

Why not serve as a salad??

SESAME-CRUSTED AUBERGINE STEAKS WITH POMEGRANATE AND WILD ROCKET

1 large or 2 medium aubergines
¼ cup olive oil
1 heaped tsp paprika
¼ cup raw honey
1 tsp Oryx desert salt
½ tsp ground black pepper
2 heaped Tbsp sesame seeds
100 g baby spinach
1 Tbsp almond flour
15 g wild rocket
80 g pomegranate arils

Cut the aubergines into steaks about 1.5 cm thick.

Combine the olive oil, paprika, honey, salt and black pepper in a large bowl.

Add the aubergine steaks and allow them to absorb the marinade. Coat the marinated aubergine steaks in the sesame seeds before cooking.

Heat a large frying pan until very hot and fry the sesame-coated aubergine steaks on both sides until golden brown.

Place the baby spinach on the bottom of a serving dish. Place the fried aubergine steaks on top, sprinkle with the almond flour and garnish with the wild rocket and pomegranate arils.

Serve immediately.

SERVINGS: 4

Ideal for meat-free Mondays served with quinoa

ROASTED PEPPER, CARAMELISED ONION AND QUINOA SALAD

3–4 bell peppers of varying colours, deseeded and cut into wedges
2 Tbsp olive oil
2 Tbsp raw honey
Oryx desert salt
¼ tsp ground black pepper
2 tsp sesame seeds
2 large red onions, diced
2 cups quinoa
1 tsp dried parsley
100 g baby spinach
1 Tbsp almond flour
chopped fresh rosemary for garnishing

1. Preheat the oven to 200 °C and spray a baking tray with non-stick cooking spray.
2. Place the bell peppers on the tray, drizzle with 1 Tbsp of the olive oil and 1 Tbsp of the honey, season with ½ tsp salt and the black pepper, and sprinkle over the sesame seeds. Roast for 30 minutes.
3. In the meantime, heat the remaining olive oil in a frying pan and fry the onions until golden brown. Drizzle with the remaining honey and season with 1 tsp salt and allow to caramelise over medium heat.
4. Cook the quinoa as per the packet instructions and season with ¼ tsp salt and the dried parsley.
5. To assemble the salad, place the quinoa in a serving bowl with the baby spinach, top with the roasted peppers and caramelised onions, and sprinkle with the almond flour. Garnish with chopped fresh rosemary before serving.

SERVINGS: 6–8

Another meat-free Monday option :-D
Serve with oven-roasted butternut wedges
(see page 145) ... mmm, delish!!!

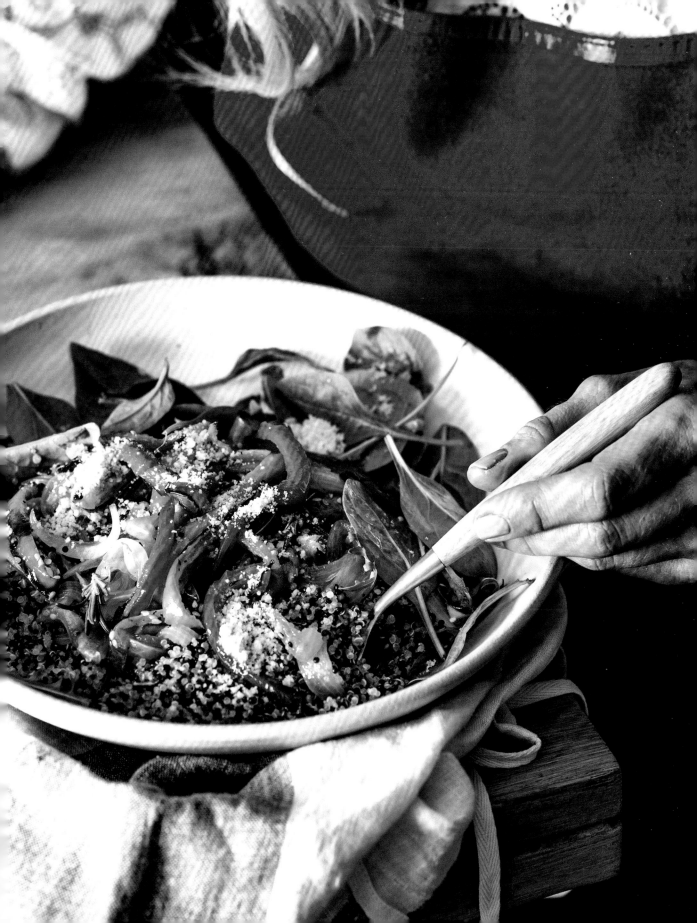

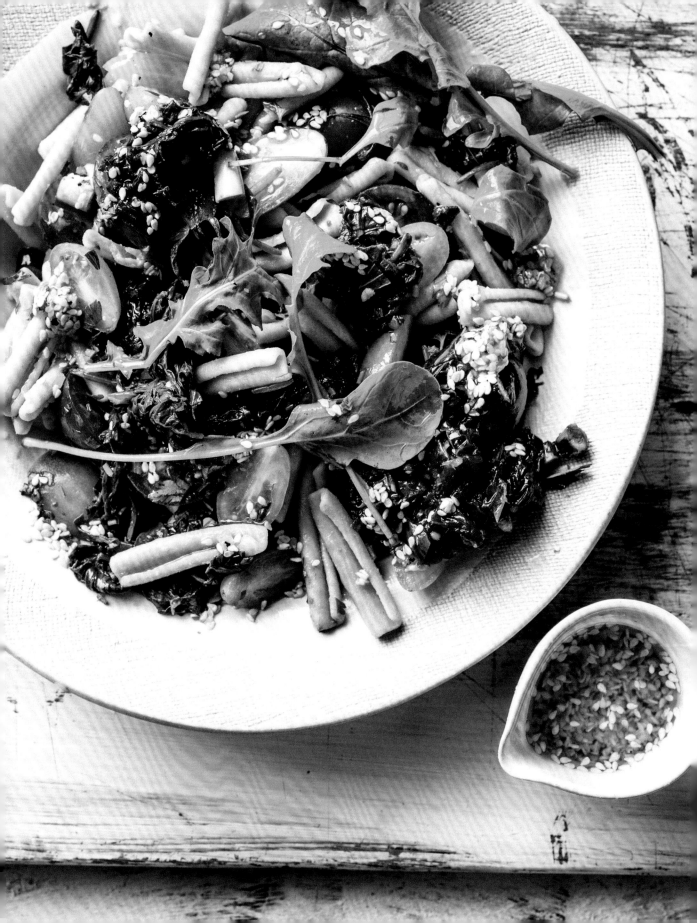

A FAVOURITE!!!

EXOTIC TOMATO AND CHICKPEA PASTA SALAD

250 g chickpea pasta
150 g baby spinach
600 g small exotic or multicoloured tomatoes, halved
8 red salad onions/scallions, chopped (leaves included)
120 g sundried tomatoes, chopped
handful chopped fresh parsley
30 g wild rocket
50 g diced or flaked almonds
fresh micro herbs for garnishing

DRESSING
1 heaped tsp crushed garlic
2 tsp Oryx desert salt
1 tsp ground black pepper
5 Tbsp olive oil
2 Tbsp raw honey
3 Tbsp sesame seeds

Cook the pasta as per the packet instructions. Drain and allow to cool. Place the baby spinach in a large mixing bowl and pour hot water over it. Set aside for 5–10 minutes to wilt, then drain well, chop and return to the bowl.

Add the tomatoes, onions, sundried tomatoes, parsley and rocket to the spinach.

Combine the dressing ingredients in a small bowl, mixing well until the honey dissolves, then pour over the salad. Add the pasta and almonds and mix well.

Garnish with micro herbs and refrigerate until needed. This is best served after 2 days.

NOTE: *Add stir-fried chicken or beef strips for a complete meal, or a handful of pumpkin seeds as a plant-based protein option.*
If you can't find chickpea pasta, you can use rice pasta instead.

SERVINGS: 6–8

Mother-in-law will approve :-D

OVEN-ROASTED STUFFED BUTTERNUT WITH WALNUTS AND CRANBERRIES

1 large or 2 medium butternuts
1 tsp olive oil
1 large red onion, diced
50 g carrot, diced
50 g celery, diced
125 g cooked brown basmati rice
handful chopped fresh thyme
1 tsp dried sage
1 tsp onion powder
100 g dried cranberries
100 g walnuts
2 Tbsp olive oil
2 Tbsp raw honey
2 Tbsp balsamic vinegar
1 Tbsp Oryx desert salt
1 tsp ground black pepper
almond flour for dusting
fresh rosemary for garnishing

1. Preheat the oven to 200 °C and spray a baking tray with non-stick cooking spray.
2. Cut the butternuts in half and remove the seeds, reserving them for later. Place the butternut halves on the baking tray and bake for 45 minutes.
3. Allow to cool slightly and then scoop out some of the flesh to create more space for the stuffing. Keep this butternut flesh.
4. Heat the oil in a frying pan and fry the onion, carrot and celery until cooked.
5. Add the butternut flesh along with the rest of the ingredients, except the almond flour and rosemary, to the pan and mix well.
6. Scoop the stuffing into the butternut halves, scatter over the reserved butternut seeds and bake for another 10 minutes.
7. Dust with almond flour and garnish with fresh rosemary before serving.

SERVINGS: 4

Makes a perfect vegetarian meal on its own, or can be served as an accompaniment to a protein of your choice

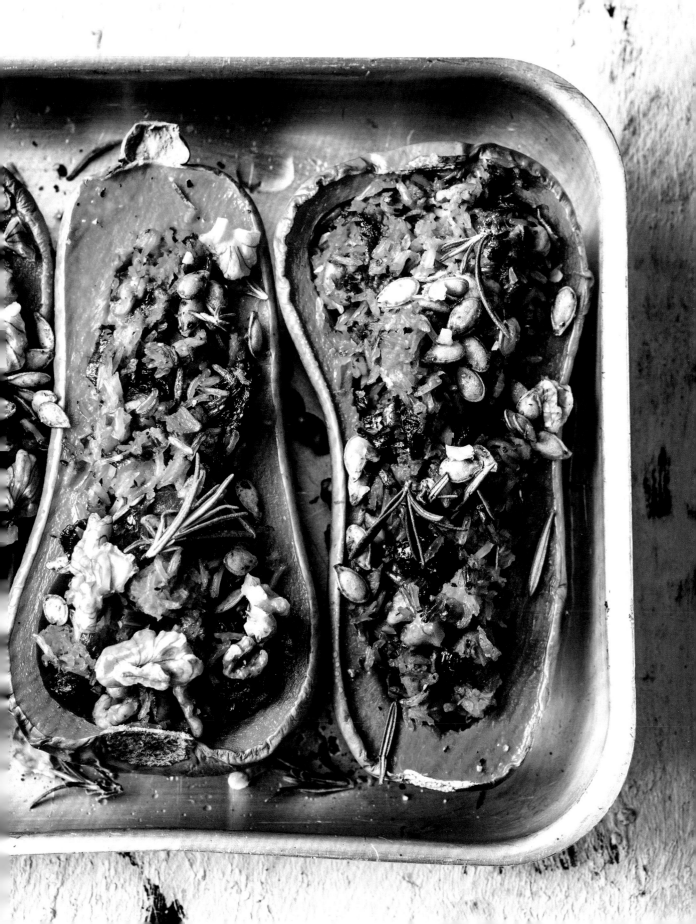

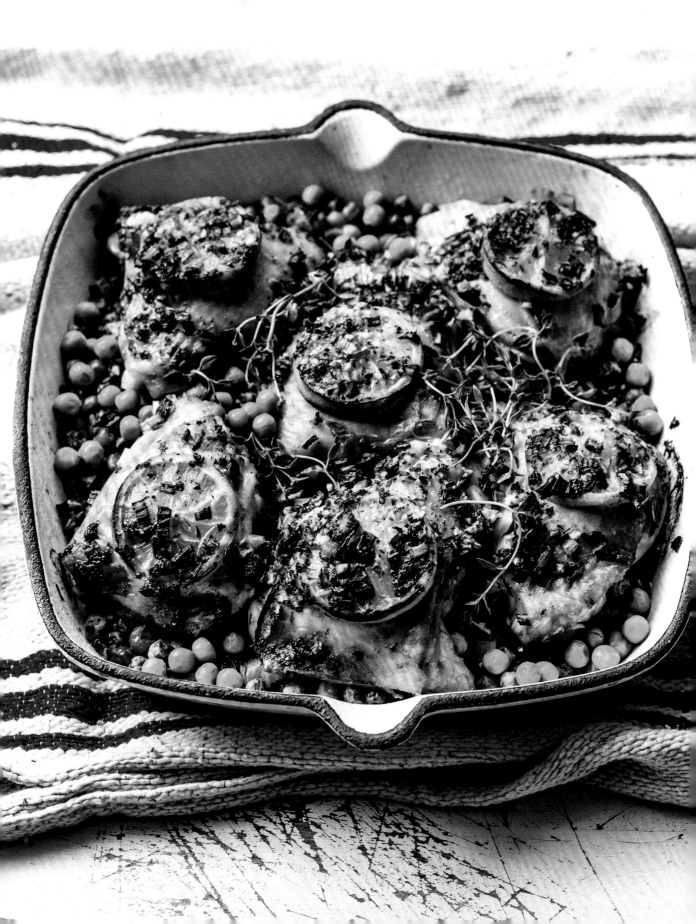

Green beans work here too

LEMON AND GARLIC GLAZED CHICKEN THIGHS WITH PEAS

500 g frozen peas
1 large red onion, diced
6 chicken thighs
6 lemon slices
2 Tbsp olive oil
1 tsp Oryx desert salt
1 tsp ground black pepper
1 tsp dried parsley
1 heaped tsp crushed garlic
2 Tbsp raw honey
juice of 2 lemons
handful of chopped fresh parsley,
thyme or baby pea shoots
for garnishing

Preheat the oven to 200 °C and spray an ovenproof dish with non-stick cooking spray.

Place the frozen peas in the bottom of the dish and add about half of the onion.

Place the chicken thighs on top of the peas and onion and place a slice of lemon on every piece of chicken.

Sprinkle the rest of the onion over the chicken.

Mix the olive oil, salt, pepper, dried parsley, garlic, honey and lemon juice in a small bowl, and then pour over the chicken.

Cover the dish with foil and bake for 15 minutes, then remove the foil and bake uncovered for another 30 minutes or until the chicken is cooked.

Garnish with chopped fresh parsley, thyme or baby pea shoots before serving with basmati rice and vegetables of your choice.

SERVINGS: 2–3

Impressive dish with minimum effort!
#you'rewelcome

FESTIVE ROAST

2 kg topside roast
150 g dried apricots
200 g dried peaches
75 g whole red salad onions/scallions, chopped (leaves included)
4 small white onions, chopped
olive oil for drizzling
2 Tbsp balsamic vinegar
¼ tsp Oryx desert wine salt
½ tsp paprika
3 whole garlic bulbs
coarse Oryx desert salt
1½ cups hot water
¼ cup raw honey
fresh rosemary for garnishing

1. Remove the roast from the fridge 30 minutes before cooking to come up to room temperature.
2. Soak the dried apricots and peaches in cold water for 30 minutes before using.
3. Preheat the oven to 200 °C on thermo-fan and spray a large roasting tray with non-stick cooking spray.
4. Pile the red and white onions, apricots and peaches in the middle of the roasting tray and drizzle with olive oil.
5. Prepare the meat by drizzling with olive oil and 1 Tbsp of the balsamic vinegar, and seasoning with the wine salt and ¼ tsp of the paprika.
6. Place the roast on top of the onions, apricots and peaches.
7. Cut the garlic bulbs in half horizontally, drizzle with olive oil and season with coarse salt. Add to the roasting tray.
8. Roast for 20 minutes, then reduce the temperature to 170 °C and roast for another hour (or 15 minutes per 500 g for medium-rare). You can cover the roast with foil once you are happy with the colour. The meat will continue to cook once removed from the oven to be medium when served.
9. Remove the roast, place on a clean tray and cover with foil. Let it rest for about 20 minutes before carving. This will give you enough time to prepare the chunky peach and apricot gravy.
10. Remove the garlic from the roasting tray and set aside. You will serve this with the roast.
11. Add the hot water, honey and remaining balsamic vinegar to the roasting tray and deglaze over low heat by stirring in all the caramelised juices, peaches and apricots. Season with coarse salt and the remaining paprika.
12. Bring to a simmer and stir occasionally until the gravy thickens.
13. Carve the roast and serve with the gravy and roast garlic and vegetable sides of your choice. Garnish with fresh rosemary.

SERVINGS: 6–8

'Deglazing' involves adding liquid to a hot pan so that you can scrape up those flavoursome browned bits of food that stick to the bottom and make oh-so-tasty gravy #you'rewelcome

HONEY AND ALMOND LONG-STEM BROCCOLI

400 g pkt long-stem broccoli
1 Tbsp olive oil
1 Tbsp raw honey
½ tsp Oryx desert salt
¼ tsp ground black pepper
25 g flaked almonds
chopped fresh parsley for garnishing

Cut a corner off the packet of broccoli and microwave on high for
6 minutes.
Heat the oil in a large frying pan and stir-fry the steamed broccoli for
4–5 minutes.
Stir through the honey, salt, black pepper and flaked almonds.
Serve warm, garnished with chopped fresh parsley.

NOTE: *This recipe works with asparagus as well as with baby or
young carrots. If using carrots, garnish with fresh thyme
instead of parsley.*

SERVINGS: 4

*All-time favourite side for its
alkalising properties*

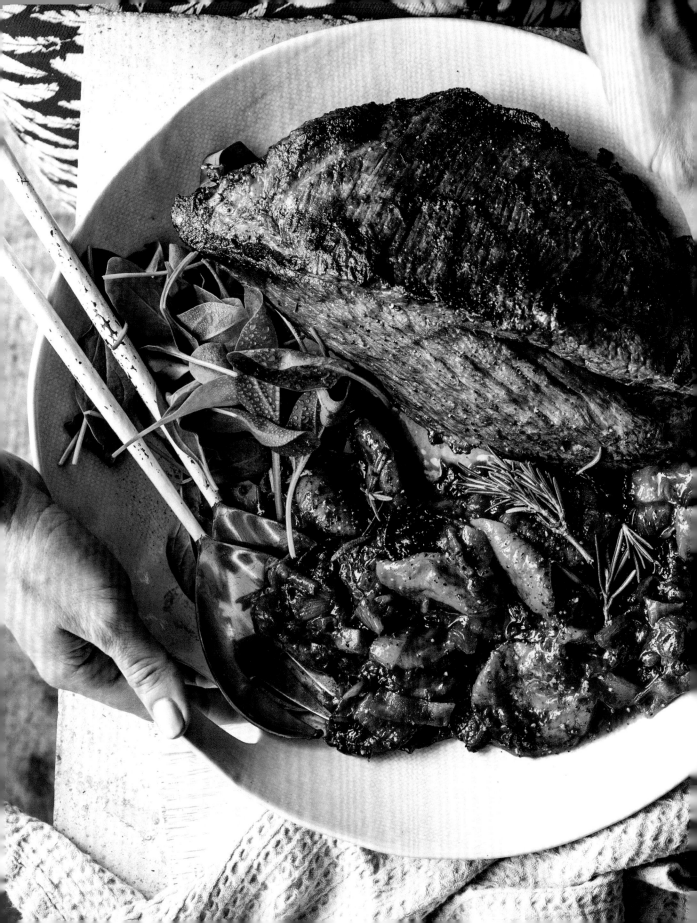

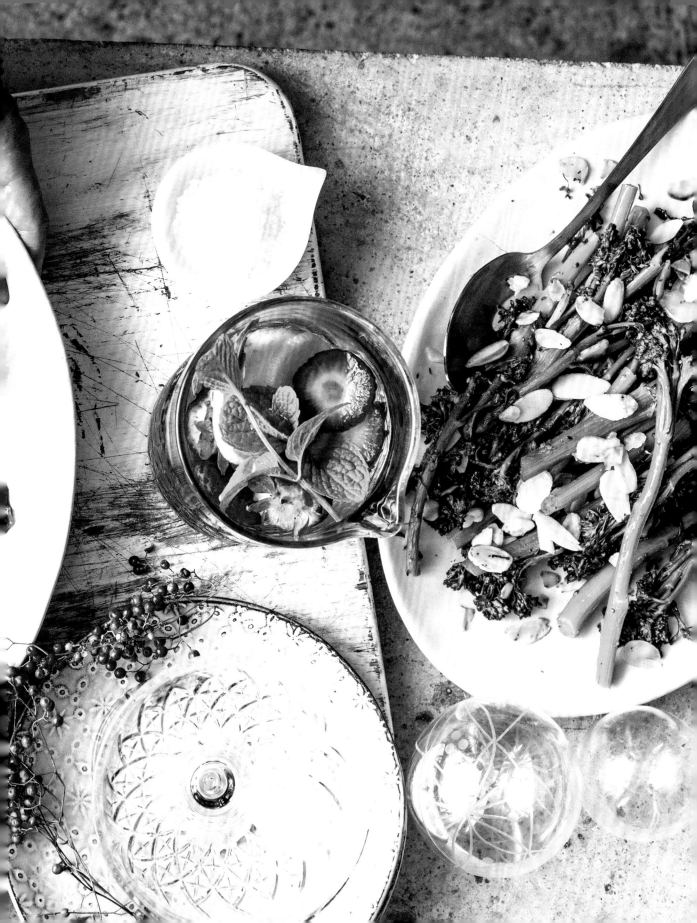

SALTED CARAMEL DATE AND PECAN PIE OR TARTLETS

CRUST

250 g almond flour
2 Tbsp raw honey
1 Tbsp water
1 tsp Oryx desert salt
1 tsp caramel essence

FILLING

600 g fresh pitted Medjool dates
2 cups hot water
4 tsp caramel essence
2 tsp vanilla essence
2 tsp Oryx desert salt
½ tsp ground cinnamon
½ tsp ground nutmeg
1 heaped Tbsp almond butter
300 g whole pecan nuts

TOPPING

crushed pecan nuts
chopped dates
almond flour
ground cinnamon

1. Preheat the oven to 200 °C. Spray a 23 cm pie dish or 6–8 loose-bottomed mini tart tins with non-stick cooking spray.
2. Combine all the ingredients for the crust in a mixing bowl, then tip into the pie dish or divide between the mini tart tins, spread out evenly and press down firmly.
3. Spray a large saucepan with non-stick cooking spray and place over medium heat.
4. Add the dates, hot water, caramel essence, vanilla essence, salt, cinnamon and nutmeg. Cook until the dates are soft and most of the water has evaporated. Remove from the heat, mash to an even texture and stir in the almond butter. Lastly, mix in the pecan nuts. (You can decide if you want to break up the pecan nuts into smaller pieces or keep them whole.)
5. Spoon the filling into the pie crust(s) and spread out evenly.
6. Top with crushed pecan nuts, chopped dates, almond flour and cinnamon before baking for 20 minutes.
7. Allow to cool before refrigerating. This is best served after a day in the fridge.

SERVINGS: 6–8

Show-stopper of NOTE!!!

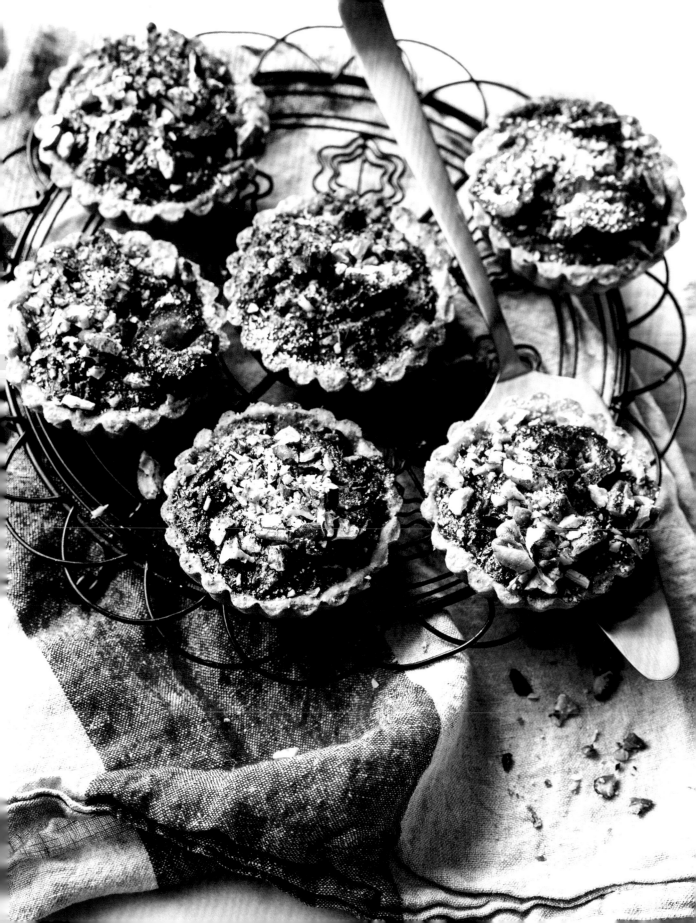

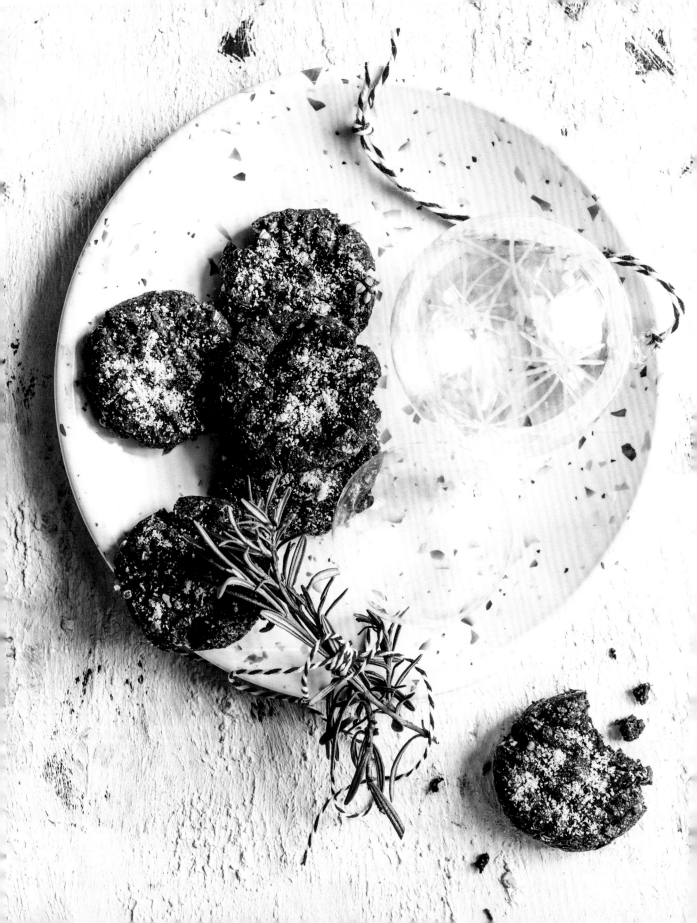

Tastes like festive family time xxx

FESTIVE BISCUITS

300 g pitted dates, chopped
300 g raisins
150 g almond flour, plus extra
for sprinkling
1 Tbsp caramel essence
1 heaped Tbsp raw cacao powder
¼ tsp ground cinnamon, plus extra
for dusting fork
¼ tsp ground nutmeg
¼ tsp ground allspice
¼ tsp Oryx desert salt
2 heaped Tbsp almond butter
150 g buckwheat
raw honey for drizzling

Soak the chopped dates and raisins in enough hot water to cover for 10–15 minutes. Drain well and mash in a large mixing bowl.

Add the rest of the ingredients, except the honey, and mix well with your hands. To prevent the mixture sticking to your hands, spray your hands with non-stick cooking spray. Once they start to get sticky, wash your hands and spray again.

Place the mixture in the fridge until completely cool.

Preheat the oven to 190 °C. Spray a baking tray with non-stick cooking spray and sprinkle with almond flour.

When you're ready, spray your hands with non-stick cooking spray and start rolling the mixture into small balls (about a heaped teaspoon per ball).

Place the balls on the prepared tray. Dip a fork in ground cinnamon and use it to gently flatten the balls into biscuits. The cinnamon will ensure that the mixture doesn't stick to the fork.

Bake for 10 minutes, then remove from the oven and immediately drizzle the biscuits with honey and sprinkle with almond flour.

Allow to cool before storing in an airtight container.

SERVINGS: 20–24 BISCUITS

Perfect with your favourite hot beverage!

INDEX